Workbook for

EMT Prehospital Care

Workbook for

EMT Prehospital Care

Fourth Edition

Eric Niegelberg, MS, NREMTP
Department of Emergency Medicine
School of Medicine
Stony Brook University
Stony Brook, New York

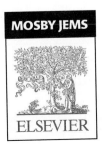

MOSBY JEMS

ELSEVIER

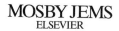
MOSBY JEMS
ELSEVIER

11830 Westline Industrial Drive
St. Louis, Missouri 63146

Workbook for EMT Prehospital Care   ISBN: 978-0-323-05505-5

ISBN 978-0-323-05505-5

Vice President and Publisher: Andrew Allen
Executive Editor: Linda Honeycutt
Developmental Editor: Kathleen Sartori
Publishing Services Manager: Patricia Tannian
Senior Project Manager: Sarah Wunderly
Design Direction: Amy Buxton

Printed in the United States

Last digit is the print number: 9   8   7   6   5   4   3   2   1

Preface

This student workbook was developed to be a learning and reinforcement tool for use by the EMT. The material in this workbook reinforces the concepts presented in the fourth edition of *EMT Prehospital Care*.

Each chapter in the workbook corresponds to a chapter in the textbook. Before completing the workbook, read the corresponding chapter in the textbook and attend the classroom session in which the chapter material is presented to you. When you complete the workbook, you should allow sufficient time to properly read each question and choose the most correct answer.

After you have completed the chapter in the workbook, use the answer key at the end of the workbook to grade yourself and to identify any areas that require further study. The answers to all of the questions in the workbook can be found in the textbook.

As an EMT, you will be working in an ever-changing environment that can be both challenging and rewarding. Each chapter in the workbook contains brief scenarios that allow you to "put it all together." These scenarios require that you identify the treatment order and priority for simulated patients. This allows you to think as a "street EMT" who is responsible for the complete care of patients. Added features in this workbook are challenging crossword puzzles and skill exercises that will vary your study experience.

This workbook contains questions that cover all of the cognitive objectives in the *National Standard Curriculum for the EMT-Basic* and the new *National Education Standards*. These are the objectives that involve knowledge and analytical skills. Throughout your EMT class, you will also be exposed to a multitude of psychomotor, or hands-on, practical skills.

Although this workbook contains multiple-choice, fill-in-the-blank, matching, and true-false questions, the certification examination may contain only multiple-choice questions. When you sit for the certification examination, you should observe the following guidelines:

- Prepare well in the weeks leading up to the test. Do not cram the night before the test. This workbook is a critical preparation tool that will instill confidence; use it.
- Get a good night's sleep the night before the exam so that you are alert and in a state of readiness to focus on the exam items.
- Eat a good meal the day of the exam to optimize your concentration abilities.
- Read each item carefully and make your selection.
- Guess the right answer before looking at the choices. This will lead you to the correct choice and instill confidence in your final selection.
- Do not spend excessive time on a particular question. Skip it and make sure you return later to finish unanswered questions. Often an answer will be found in a later question.
- Don't become overwhelmed. If you feel stressed, take a few slow breaths and refocus.

Eric Niegelberg

Contents

1 Introduction to Emergency Medical Care

MULTIPLE CHOICE

1. A system of resources and personnel necessary to provide immediate care to ill and injured persons describes a(n):
   a. Emergency medical services (EMS) system
   b. Ambulance service
   c. Enhanced 9-1-1 dispatching system
   d. Hospital emergency service

2. Most of the growth and technical development of prehospital emergency care emerged from:
   a. Disaster drills
   b. Outpatient programs
   c. War
   d. Laboratory animal research

3. The Civil War is noted for the first use in the United States of:
   a. Military antishock trousers
   b. Mobile army surgical hospital units
   c. Ambulances
   d. A formal system of triage

4. The Korean War saw the first use of:
   a. Large-bore intravenous lines to stabilize the patient in the field.
   b. Large hospital ships to provide definitive care to all patients.
   c. Physicians assigned to every platoon.
   d. Helicopters to provide rapid transport of casualties.

5. Michael Reese Hospital in Chicago is credited with the first use of:
   a. Horse-drawn ambulances
   b. Motorized ambulances
   c. Military antishock trousers
   d. Emergency medical technicians (EMTs)

6. Trauma is the leading cause of death in the age group of:
   a. 1 to 45 years
   b. 45 to 50 years
   c. 50 to 60 years
   d. Over 60 years

7. The National Academy of Sciences published a landmark paper entitled "Accidental Death and Disability: the Neglected Disease of Modern Society" in:
   a. 1966
   b. 1970
   c. 1945
   d. 1973

8. Ambulances, medical direction, human resources, evaluation, and hospitals are all components of a(n):
   a. EMS system
   b. Health care agency
   c. Emergency network
   d. Crisis intervention team

9. The hospital's emergency department (ED), which is a component of an EMS system, is the "intersection of care" for the critical patient because the ED:
   a. Provides definitive care to a patient before discharge.
   b. Trains the public in cardiopulmonary resuscitation (CPR) and first aid.
   c. Provides stabilizing measures to prehospital patients before transfer to the operating room or critical care unit.
   d. Coordinates multiple components of every EMS system.

10. The lay rescuer is someone who:
    a. Is not a part of the EMS system.
    b. Can never provide CPR and first aid for the patient.
    c. Treats the patient in the emergency department.
    d. Is often the first to help the patient.

11. _____ is a method of hospital designation and an essential part of an EMS system that uses capabilities in different areas of care such as trauma, burns, neonatology, and replantation.
    a. Specialty referral center
    b. Standardization
    c. Systemization
    d. Alteration

12. This aspect of an EMS system brings to the scene the first medical personnel that patients are likely to encounter. These individuals may use either basic or advanced skills to support and stabilize the critical patient:
    a. Lay rescuer
    b. Emergency departments
    c. Emergency medical responders
    d. Intensive care units

13. Physician involvement and participation in all phases of the EMS system to ensure quality care best define the concept of:
    a. Categorization
    b. Standardization
    c. Systemization
    d. Medical direction

14. Patient assessment, patient care, and transfer of the patient to hospital staff are:
    a. Beyond the scope of practice of the EMT.
    b. Primary roles of the EMT in most systems.
    c. Acts that must be completed and documented to prevent an act of negligence.
    d. Taken together to form the basis for malfeasance.

15. "Acting requisite to the body of knowledge which defines the service and abilities of the professional ... according to the oath of the profession. Historically first applied to religious vows ...." This definition best describes the term:
    a. Competence
    b. Professionalism
    c. Ethics
    d. Honor
16. The person who usually is the first medical person to see the patient best describes the:
    a. Physician
    b. EMT-Basic
    c. Lay rescuer
    d. Nurse
17. The person who interprets the electrocardiogram, performs invasive airway skills, and has a more broadly based knowledge of pharmacology best describes the:
    a. EMT-Paramedic
    b. EMT
    c. EMT-Defibrillation
    d. First responder
18. Quality improvement programs are designed to:
    a. Provide a system of internal and external reviews.
    b. Provide immunity from liability for the EMT.
    c. Review ambulance runs and allow for continuing medical education.
    d. Both a and c.
19. The EMT:
    a. Practices medicine without medical direction.
    b. Is not responsible to physician directors.
    c. Is a designated agent of the physician.
    d. Is not responsible for quality improvement issues.
20. Running reviews, audits, and gathering feedback from patients and hospital staff are all components of:
    a. The EMT recertification process
    b. Initial EMT training
    c. Medical direction
    d. The quality improvement process
21. Speaking directly with a physician for advice, by telephone or radio from the patient's side, is known as:
    a. Offline physician control
    b. Quality improvement
    c. Medical communications
    d. Online medical direction
22. Standing orders and written protocols are all components of:
    a. Offline medical direction
    b. Online medical control
    c. Physician control
    d. Hospital direction
23. The first link in the American Heart Association's "chain of survival" is:
    a. EMT training courses
    b. Early 9-1-1 access
    c. CPR
    d. Defibrillation

MATCHING

Questions 24-28. Indicate which of the roles of the EMT listed in column A are primary versus secondary (other) in most systems. Column B items can be used more than once.

Column A	**Column B**
24. _____ Patient assessment	a. Primary
25. _____ Extrication	b. Secondary (other)
26. _____ Personal safety and safety of others	
27. _____ Transfer of the patient to hospital staff	
28. _____ Lifting and moving of patients	

Questions 29-32. Match the appropriate personal protective equipment in column B with the potential hazard in column A.

Column A	**Column B**
29. _____ Bandaging a minor bleeding wound	a. Gloves
30. _____ Bandaging a spurting wound	b. Goggles
31. _____ Suctioning a patient's airway	c. Both a and b
32. _____ Emergency childbirth	d. Neither a nor b

FILL IN THE BLANK

33. The _____ _____ provides initial care such as CPR to the patient with minimal equipment before the arrival of the ambulance.

34. The _____ system is responsible for notification, prioritization of calls, and dispatch.

35. _____ is equipment that allows for the transmission of ECG data from the patient in the field to the physician at the base hospital.

SHORT ANSWER

36. List six methods that the EMT may use as part of his or her role in quality improvement.

    a. _____
    _____
    _____
    _____

    b. _____
    _____
    _____
    _____

c. _____
_____
_____

d. _____
_____
_____

e. _____
_____
_____

f. _____
_____
_____

TRUE/FALSE

37. _____ Documenting all aspects of prehospital care on a call report is an essential aspect of protection against lawsuits.

38. _____ Effective communication with a family member at the scene of an incident is not an important role for the EMT because the hospital staff is responsible for keeping the family informed about the status of the patient.

39. _____ The National Registry of Emergency Medical Technicians was developed to standardize treatment protocols on a national level.

40. _____ The American Heart Association establishes standards and guidelines for emergency cardiac care for both hospital and prehospital care providers.

CASE SCENARIO

Questions 41 to 43 refer to the following scenario.
You receive a call to respond to a motor vehicle crash at the intersection of Main Street and Washington Avenue. When you arrive, you find a single car that struck a utility pole, with minor damage to the front end. You determine that there was only one person in the car, and this driver is sitting on the curb. A bystander is applying direct pressure to a minor laceration on the patient's thigh. The patient tells you that he does not want to go to the hospital. After taking a complete set of vital signs, you call your base physician, who speaks directly to the patient in an attempt to convince him to go to the hospital.

41. The bystander that began treatment of the patient before your arrival can be classified as a(n):
   a. Lay rescuer
   b. Technician
   c. EMT
   d. Paramedic

42. The contact that you make with medical control is considered _____ medical control.

43. The appropriate personal protection devices to use when bandaging this patient's wound are:
   a. Disposable medical gloves, goggles, and a gown
   b. Disposable medical gloves and goggles
   c. Goggles and a face mask
   d. Disposable medical gloves

CROSSWORD PUZZLE

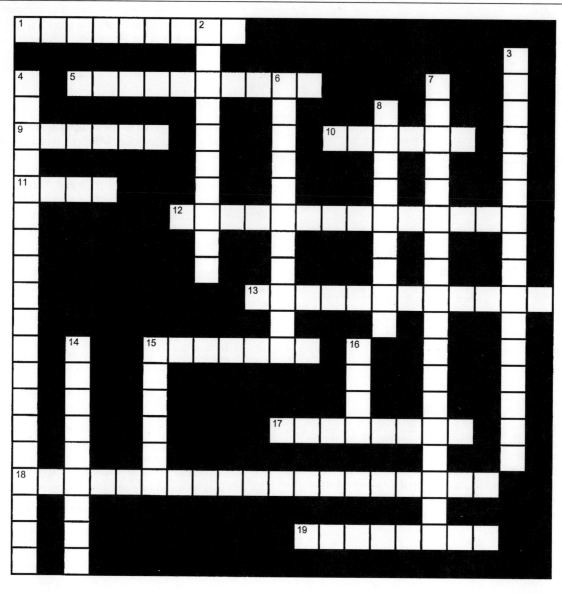

Across

1. Serves as team leader for in-hospital and prehospital personnel
5. Bystander who provides initial first aid to a victim
9. Sorting according to medical need
10. Helicopters were first used to evacuate the wounded during this war
11. Military hospitals are referred to as _____ units
12. Facility that provides online medical direction
13. Transmission of patient data by radio or telephone
15. _____ medical direction is medical guidance in the form of written protocols
17. _____ 9-1-1 allows the dispatcher to track the caller's exact location
18. Serves as the intersection of care in the EMS system
19. System through which emergency vehicles are summoned to respond

Down

2. Systematic collection and analysis of information obtained through examination
3. The physician's responsibility for the medical conduct of EMS personnel
4. Leading cause of trauma deaths
6. Process by which entrapped patients are rescued
7. System of reviews and audits of all aspects of an EMS system
8. Written policies or procedures that delineate patient care
14. Highest level of training for EMS workers
15. _____ medical direction involves real-time contact with a physician
16. Type of mask worn when treating a patient with suspected tuberculosis

4

2 Well-Being of the EMT

MULTIPLE CHOICE

1. Which of the following emotional reactions is common for the EMT to experience when dealing with death, dying, and illness?
   a. Loss of appetite
   b. Feelings of success
   c. Feeling appreciated
   d. Increased appetite

2. Emotions of guilt, grief, anger, loss of appetite, and increased alcohol or drug use experienced by the EMT are related to:
   a. Pain
   b. Organic illness
   c. Warning signs of stress
   d. Phobias

3. When a family member wants to view the body of a deceased loved one, you should:
   a. Encourage them to avoid this to prevent hysterical reactions.
   b. Tell them that they can view the body at a later time.
   c. Allow them to view the body.
   d. Make them wait until the physician arrives.

4. When dealing with the family of a patient who has just died, the EMT should:
   a. Attend strictly to the patient's needs.
   b. Be supportive and nonjudgmental.
   c. Point out to the family that they should have called EMS sooner.
   d. Leave the scene because your services are not required.

5. When arriving at the scene, the EMT should:
   a. Disregard the family member if he or she does not need medical attention.
   b. Ask the family about the patient's condition.
   c. Ignore the family member because he or she is not the patient.
   d. Not acknowledge the family member's concern about his or her loved one.

6. Which of the following represents an emotion that may be experienced by a family member of the EMT?
   a. A complete understanding of the EMT's work
   b. No fear of being ignored or left out
   c. No feelings of competition with the job
   d. Resentment and feelings of being left out

7. To fulfill a commitment to his or her family, the EMT should:
   a. Overlook the needs of loved ones.
   b. Organize a work schedule to include time for family needs.
   c. Keep experiences inside because family members will not understand.
   d. Separate work and family for the family's benefit.

8. A simple approach that the EMT can exercise when faced with a particularly stressful incident, such as the death of a child, is to:
   a. Share the feelings with a colleague or a family member.
   b. Take a strict clinical approach to avoid such feelings.
   c. Ignore it through positive thinking.
   d. Not think about it to avoid the stress.

9. A sense of hopelessness, loss of appetite, and feelings of isolation are all signs of:
   a. Debriefing sickness
   b. Psychological emergencies
   c. Denial
   d. Stress induced by job-related activities

10. Major disasters such as the death of a child may require a more organized response by the EMT to resolve negative feelings. This process is called a(n):
    a. Critical incident stress debriefing
    b. Encounter group
    c. Catharsis
    d. Exchange session

11. The primary reason an EMT is responsible for scene safety is because:
    a. The patient may have sustained additional injury.
    b. The patient has already sustained enough.
    c. The family may take legal action against you.
    d. The EMT is trained in safety procedures for self and others at the scene.

12. The EMT is faced with hazards that include communicable disease, hazardous materials, and personal threats of violence. The first way the EMT can protect himself or herself after arriving at the scene is to:
    a. Perform an initial assessment.
    b. Call for backup assistance.
    c. Perform a scene safety size-up.
    d. Use community resources.

13. Body substance isolation (standard precautions) considers:
    a. All body fluids from all patients as potentially infectious.
    b. Blood from sick patients as potentially infectious.
    c. Blood from high-risk patients as potentially infectious.
    d. All body fluids from patients with HIV as potentially infectious.

14. When confronted with an open wound oozing blood, the EMT should:
    a. Avoid the patient, only touching as necessary.
    b. Wipe the blood with a sterile bandage.
    c. Put on disposable medical gloves before treating the patient.
    d. Place a surgical face mask on the patient.
15. Diseases capable of being spread from one person to another are called:
    a. Communicable
    b. Endocrine
    c. Genetic
    d. Syndromes
16. Standard precautions are used with:
    a. Patients with AIDS
    b. All patients
    c. Patients with infections
    d. Patients with hepatitis
17. The routine practice of wearing protective clothing (e.g., gloves, protective eyewear) when performing certain procedures (e.g., bleeding control, airway control) is called:
    a. General infection prevention
    b. Barrier model
    c. Immunization
    d. Body substance isolation (standard precautions)
18. The simplest and most effective way to block the spread of infection is:
    a. Avoiding physical contact with patients.
    b. Using alcohol wipes on infection sites.
    c. Handwashing before and after every patient contact.
    d. Wearing a gown with every patient contact.
19. The primary responsibility of an EMT at the scene of a hazardous materials fire is:
    a. Containment
    b. Removal
    c. Decontamination
    d. Emergency medical care
20. The first priority with a potentially dangerous patient is:
    a. The patient's protection
    b. Self-protection
    c. The legal implications
    d. Restraining the patient
21. The most common cause of death for an EMT on the job is:
    a. Violence related
    b. Motor vehicle related
    c. Caused by an infectious disease
    d. Caused by terrorist activities
22. The most common cause of injury to EMS workers is (are):
    a. Injuries to the extremities
    b. Injuries caused by violence
    c. Injuries to the back
    d. Loss of hearing

MATCHING

Questions 23-26. Match the personal protective equipment in column B to the hazard in column A.

Column A	Column B
23. _____ Bleeding laceration	a. HEPA respirator
24. _____ Psychiatric emergency	b. Disposable medical gloves
25. _____ Hazardous materials scene	c. Binoculars
26. _____ Patient with tuberculosis	d. Soft restraints

FILL IN THE BLANK

27. Securing items of potential importance at a crime scene is part of the _____ _____ _____.

28. The time period in which a person can transmit an infectious disease to others is called the _____ _____.

29. The stage of dying in which patients are profoundly sad and experience immense grief is called _____.

30. The system in the body that protects against microorganisms is called the _____ system.

31. The time between contact with an infectious agent and the onset of symptoms is called the _____ _____.

32. _____ _____ is the mode of disease transmission that occurs when the EMT touches a contaminated instrument.

33. Infections are caused by _____ that are toxic to the body, such as bacteria and viruses.

34. The receptacle used for the safe disposal of used needles is a _____ _____.

35. _____ _____ that incorporate universal precautions and body substance isolation should be used in all situations to avoid transmission from both recognized and unrecognized sources of infection.

36. _____ is spread by droplets and the airborne route and requires the EMT to wear a high-efficiency particulate air (HEPA) respirator mask to minimize the risk of disease transmission.

37. Transmission of disease by a tick or mosquito is called _____ _____.

38. List three features of a pandemic flu.

    a. _____   c. _____

        _____   _____

    b. _____

        _____

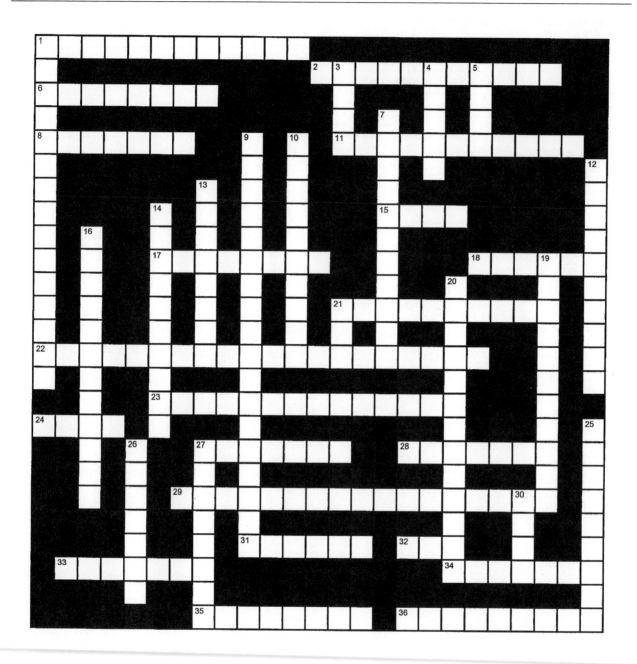

Across

1. The body's protection against microorganisms
2. The most important measure for blocking the spread of infection
6. An early intervention that occurs shortly after a disaster to stop the negative stress process
8. German measles
11. Your first concern when responding to a call
15. Government agency that sets rules regarding exposure of emergency personnel to communicable diseases in the course of their work
17. The ability to resist the development of pathogenic microorganisms or their toxic effects
18. A person who is infected with an illness that may be spread
21. Stage of dying when patients may negotiate with God to extend their life
22. Illnesses that are capable of being spread from one person to another
23. Identification and assistance of distressed emergency workers
24. A susceptible person who, if exposed to a source, may become ill
27. Free from germs
28. Type of disease transmission that occurs when an infected person coughs or sneezes
29. _____ _____ education sessions designed to familiarize emergency responders with the nature of emergency service stress
31. Term used when a patient refuses to believe the seriousness of the situation
32. Government agency that creates guidelines to standardize infection control practices
33. Person who shows no signs of disease, but may be a source of infection to others
34. Lockjaw
35. The coming in contact with, but not necessarily being infected by, a disease-causing agent
36. Infection of the liver caused by viruses

Down

1. Transmission of infection through a contact of the susceptible host with a contaminated intermediate object
3. Acquired immunodeficiency syndrome
4. Stage of dying when patients project irate feelings onto others
5. High-efficiency particulate air respirator used in the prevention of transmission of tuberculosis
7. Transmission of disease by means of an organism, such as tick or mosquito
9. Time period during which a person can transmit an infectious disease to others
10. Final stage of dying when patients ultimately accept the situation
12. Stage of dying when patients are profoundly sad and experience immense grief
13. A national telephone resource that provides advice on how to handle chemical emergencies
14. Varicella
16. Method by which an infectious agent travels from the source to the host
19. Rigidity of the muscles that occurs at death
20. Physical transmission of infection between a susceptible host and an infected person
21. Precaution designed to reduce the risk of transmission of pathogens from moist body substances
25. Whooping cough
26. A sign that identifies hazardous materials
27. Transmission of microorganisms carried in the air and inhaled by a susceptible host
30. Specialized mask and regulator with portable air supply used by rescue personnel in environments that might contain hazardous materials

9

3 Medicolegal and Ethical Issues

1. A serious effort to acquire the requisite skills taught in the initial EMT training program, as well as a continued effort to prevent deterioration of knowledge, is the best way to maintain:
   a. Respect
   b. Competence
   c. Certification
   d. Analytical skills

2. You have completed the treatment and transportation of a patient who sustained a gunshot wound to the chest. On leaving the hospital, you are approached by a reporter from the local newspaper. You may:
   a. Share the vital signs of the patient.
   b. Say that the patient is all right and give the reporter a copy of the ambulance call report.
   c. Refer the reporter to your supervisor or hospital officials for comment.
   d. Recount the past medical history as told to you by the patient.

3. The body of knowledge, laws, policies, standards, and guidelines set forth by various standard-setting organizations that provides the basis of prehospital care, along with the everyday practice of other providers, best describes:
   a. Values of practice
   b. The standard of care
   c. Emergency laws
   d. Competence

4. A duty to act, a breach of duty, an injury to the patient, and a causal connection between the injury and the EMT's actions are all ingredients of:
   a. Abandonment
   b. Negligence
   c. Malfeasance
   d. An emergency medical services system

5. Your ambulance is on the scene where a 72-year-old woman tripped on the curb and injured her hip. You inform her of the benefits and consequences of the care provided and she agrees to allow you to treat her. She is being treated under the concept of _____ consent.
   a. implied
   b. applied
   c. expressed (informed)
   d. presumed

6. Your ambulance is on the scene of a 54-year-old woman who is having a heart attack. During treatment of this patient, you hear another call for a child who is choking approximately 1 mile away.

If you leave your patient and respond to the child who is choking, you may be guilty of:
   a. Malfeasance
   b. Abandonment
   c. Negligence
   d. Breach of duty

7. Your ambulance is dispatched to the scene of a "man down." On arrival you find a 52-year-old unconscious patient. Treatment may be rendered under the concept of _____ consent.
   a. informed
   b. expressed
   c. implied
   d. surrogate

8. An emancipated minor is a(n):
   a. Individual who is younger than the legal adult age but who is living independently of the parent.
   b. Child who is injured at school, and the parent is at work.
   c. Patient who has been judged mentally incompetent by the court.
   d. Individual who is younger than the legal adult age but who is injured while working.

9. Good Samaritan laws are designed to protect the:
   a. EMT against legal action from abandonment of the patient.
   b. EMT against legal action from gross negligence when driving the ambulance.
   c. EMT against legal action if cardiopulmonary resuscitation (CPR) is not started on a patient in witnessed cardiac arrest and who is pronounced dead at the scene.
   d. Any person who is functioning in a nonprofessional capacity and without an expectation of remuneration.

10. If an EMT observes a person removing evidence from a crime scene, the EMT should:
   a. Report it to police and document the event.
   b. Ignore it because that is the role of the police, not the EMT.
   c. Investigate the issue carefully before making a decision.
   d. Retrieve the object from the individual and place it in its original location.

11. A patient's willingness to donate his or her organs is usually documented on a:
   a. Passport
   b. DNR order
   c. Driver's license
   d. Social Security card

12. Deviation from the accepted standard of care that results in the injury of a patient best describes:
    a. Malpractice
    b. An ethical breach
    c. Nonfeasance
    d. Battery
13. An alert, adult patient complaining of chest pain is refusing medical care. You should first:
    a. Have the patient sign a release form.
    b. Try to convince the patient to go to the hospital.
    c. Place the patient on the stretcher and transport.
    d. Advise the patient to call again if the pain becomes worse.
14. Good Samaritan legislation:
    a. Is only applicable in approximately 25% of the United States.
    b. Alleviates the need for the EMT to be concerned about his or her actions.
    c. Is intended to encourage people to help others without fear of litigation when emergencies arise.
    d. Only protects you when you are a paid emergency medical services professional while at work.
15. You are treating a 27-year-old man who was the target of a drive-by shooting. The patient sustained a gunshot wound to the left upper leg. The police are concerned that all evidence be optimally preserved. Your actions would include:
    a. Do not remove the patient's pants because the bullet hole is evidence.
    b. Remove or cut the pants, but try to avoid cutting through the bullet hole.
    c. Do not be concerned with the patient's clothing because this is not considered evidence.
    d. Only transport the patient after the police crime scene unit has photographed the patient's wounds.

FILL IN THE BLANK

16. The guiding standard of effective medical practice is referred to as the _____ _____ _____.

17. Physical contact with a person without his or her consent and without legal justification is known as _____.

SHORT ANSWER

18. List the four elements that must be proved for negligence to exist.
    _____
    _____

_____
_____
_____
_____
_____
_____

CASE SCENARIOS

19. You are called to the scene at a restaurant, where you encounter a 54-year-old female patient. According to her companion, the patient became very pale and then had a syncopal episode that lasted for about 2 minutes. The patient is now alert and is refusing any further care. Although the patient tells you her demographic information, she refuses your attempts to assess her condition, including taking vital signs. Her companion tells you that you should take the patient to the hospital, but the patient refuses. You should:
    a. Restrain the patient and transport her to the hospital.
    b. Tell the companion that there is nothing more that you can do, then leave.
    c. Explain to the patient your concerns for her welfare and state that her condition may be life threatening. If she still refuses care, contact online medical control, if available, and have your patient sign a "refusal of medical advice."
    d. Wait with the patient for 15 to 30 minutes to see if any symptoms recur; if they do not recur, leave the scene.

Questions 20 to 22 refer to the following scenario.
You respond to a scene at the shopping mall and encounter an 18-year-old woman who tripped on a loose piece of carpeting and twisted her ankle. Your evaluation reveals a swollen left ankle without any other trauma. The patient is alert and oriented and tells you that she wants to sue the store. You advise the patient that you want to take her to the hospital for further evaluation.
20. What type of consent is required before treating this patient?
    a. Implied consent is required.
    b. Informed consent is required.
    c. No consent is required because the patient is an emancipated minor.
    d. Consent can only be granted by the police because the patient intends to sue.
21. The patient agrees to be transported to the hospital, and you help her walk to the ambulance. While walking, the patient stumbles and falls to the ground, injuring her wrist. Having this patient walk, rather than immobilizing her ankle and

transporting her on a stretcher, is a deviation from:
- a. The Good Samaritan laws.
- b. The level of consent agreed to by the patient.
- c. The standard of care.
- d. Quality care (abandonment).

22. You are now en route to the hospital and have an estimated arrival time of 25 minutes. The patient has severe pain in both her ankle and her wrist. While you are working as an EMT, you have the keys to the advanced life support (ALS) cabinet in the ambulance, and you administer a pain reliever to the patient from the ALS equipment. Use of ALS equipment by an EMT is:
- a. Outside the scope of practice.
- b. Allowable under the "Golden Rule" concept.
- c. Outside the level of consent agreed to by the patient.
- d. Allowable for a volunteer EMT but not for a paid EMT.

Questions 23 and 24 refer to the following scenario.
You respond to the local nursing home and encounter an 87-year-old woman in her bed in severe respiratory distress. The nursing home tells you that the local community hospital, approximately 12 minutes away, is expecting the patient in the emergency department. In addition to a lengthy medical history, the nursing home gives you a copy of a valid DNR order that was signed by all appropriate parties 2 weeks ago. The patient is currently receiving low-flow oxygen by a nasal cannula. The patient is not able to answer any questions at this time.

23. Care for this patient en route to the hospital consists of:
- a. Removing the supplemental oxygen and providing psychological first aid and transport; no interventions can be performed because of the DNR.
- b. Maintaining the oxygen as established by the personnel from the nursing home at its current level, but making no adjustments because of the DNR.
- c. Providing any needed interventions to properly treat this patient's respiratory distress, including adjusting the oxygen delivery system as required.
- d. Only providing specific care if the patient has a health care proxy present.

24. You are approximately 3 minutes from the hospital when the patient stops breathing. You should:
- a. Begin positive-pressure ventilation by mouth to mouth or some other adjunct.
- b. Continue to monitor the patient, but not provide positive-pressure ventilations.
- c. Return the patient to the nursing home, because no care can be rendered.
- d. Begin CPR.

Chapter **3** **Medicolegal and Ethical Issues**

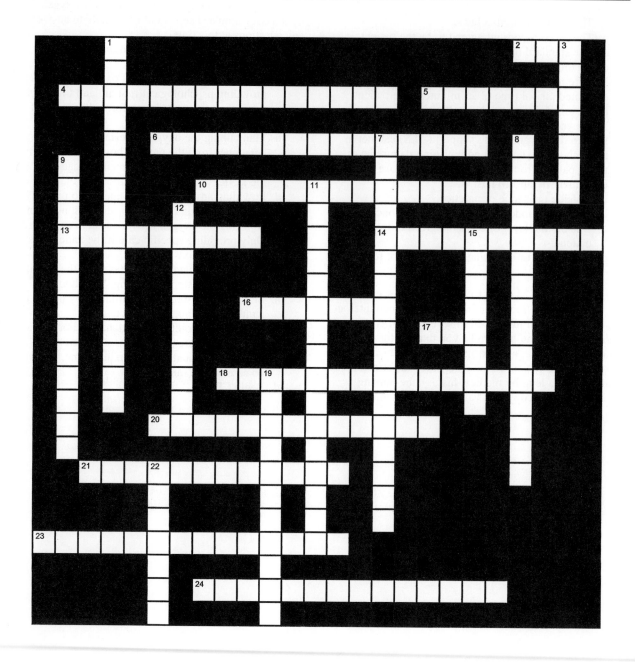

Chapter **3** **Medicolegal and Ethical Issues**   Copyright © 2010, 2007, 2004, 1997, 1992 by Mosby, Inc., an affiliate of Elsevier Inc. All rights reserved.

Across

2. Committee that approves research studies
4. A person who is legally able to make medical decisions for a patient who is incapacitated
5. Permission to medically treat
6. Maintaining a patient's right to privacy
10. Process by which an emotionally disturbed or incompetent patient who is a danger to self or others is moved to a medical facility by police and emergency personnel
13. The legal requirement to evaluate and treat a patient
14. Deviation from the accepted standard of care resulting in injury to the patient
16. Consent to medically treat an unconscious patient
17. Orders directing health care providers not to provide CPR
18. The process of securing items of potential importance at a crime scene
20. A brand of bracelet or necklace that indicates a preexisting medical condition
21. Negligent act or omission that violates the standards of care expected
23. Practices by health care providers that reduce the possibility of a lawsuit
24. Guiding rule of effective medical practice

Down

1. Individual who is younger than the legal adult age but who is legally allowed to give consent because he or she is married
3. Offensive touching or use of force on a person
7. Specific statements of instruction regarding care that a patient does or does not want performed, should he or she become incapacitated
8. Parameters and limitations of a medical provider
9. Laws designed to protect the private citizen who is functioning in a nonprofessional capacity and without an expectation of remuneration
11. Clear connection between the patient's injury and actions taken or omitted by the EMT (an element that must be present to prove negligence)
12. "Do unto others as you would have them do unto you"
15. Consent to medically treat, after providing the patient with knowledge of the steps and procedures and related risks
19. An EMT who prematurely leaves a patient in need of emergency care and transportation to a hospital is subject to a charge of _____
22. A threat or attempt to inflict bodily harm on a person

4 The Human Body

MULTIPLE CHOICE

1. The study of the structure or form of living things is called:
   a. Anatomy
   b. Physics
   c. Biology
   d. Physiology

2. Which of the following is a function of the skeletal system?
   a. Gives structure and support
   b. Produces plasma
   c. Destroys red blood cells
   d. Initiates respiration

3. In the normal anatomic position, the body is erect with feet together and parallel, arms extended, and palms and head facing:
   a. Medially
   b. Posteriorly
   c. Anteriorly
   d. Laterally

4. The heart, great vessels, esophagus, and trachea are located in which of the following body spaces?
   a. Pleura
   b. Peritoneal cavity
   c. Mediastinum
   d. Pelvic cavity

5. The ilium, ischium and pubis collectively form the:
   a. Shoulder girdle
   b. Pelvic girdle
   c. Thoracic cage
   d. Metacarpal bones

6. The abdominal quadrants are created by two intersecting lines that meet at the:
   a. Xiphoid process
   b. Epigastric region
   c. Umbilicus
   d. Pubic bone

7. The respiratory structure responsible for preventing aspiration of food and other materials into the airway is called the:
   a. Bronchiole
   b. Carina
   c. Pharynx
   d. Epiglottis

8. The movement of oxygen from the lungs to the blood occurs at the level of the:
   a. Bronchi
   b. Alveoli
   c. Trachea
   d. Larynx

9. The pumping chambers of the heart that deliver blood to the lungs and body tissues are called the:
   a. Septums
   b. Sinuses
   c. Atria
   d. Ventricles

10. The major artery that delivers blood to the body or systemic circulation is called the:
    a. Aorta
    b. Pulmonary artery
    c. Coronary artery
    d. Vena cava

11. The type of vessel that permits diffusion to take place and that is one cell thick is called a(n):
    a. Capillary
    b. Vein
    c. Arteriole
    d. Artery

12. The type of blood cell that is responsible for combating infection is called:
    a. Red blood cell
    b. White blood cell
    c. Platelet
    d. Plasma

13. The protein that is responsible for the transport of oxygen and carbon dioxide is called:
    a. Plasma
    b. Thrombin
    c. Hemoglobin
    d. Fibrinogen

14. Which of the following is part of the central nervous system?
    a. Spinal cord
    b. Brain
    c. Peripheral nerves
    d. Both a and b

15. The part of the brain responsible for balance and coordination is called the:
    a. Cerebrum
    b. Pons
    c. Medulla
    d. Cerebellum

16. The body system concerned with maintaining homeostasis and influencing growth, reproduction, and response to stress through the release of hormones is called the:
    a. Digestive system
    b. Circulatory system
    c. Endocrine system
    d. Lymphatic system

17

17. The organ responsible for the release of insulin, which allows the metabolism of glucose, is the:
    a. Liver
    b. Gallbladder
    c. Pancreas
    d. Spleen
18. The largest part of the digestive tract, where absorption of nutrients occurs, is called the:
    a. Esophagus
    b. Liver
    c. Small intestine
    d. Rectum
19. The urinary system tube responsible for transporting urine from the bladder to the external opening of both the male and the female genitalia is called the:
    a. Ureter
    b. Urethra
    c. Common bile duct
    d. Prostate
20. The tube that connects the ovary to the uterus is called the:
    a. Fallopian tube
    b. Cervix
    c. Ovarian tubule
    d. Uterine duct
21. The heart, lungs, and brain depend on one another to maintain vital functions. Which of the following reasons best explains why a patient stops breathing after a cardiac arrest?
    a. Lack of oxygen to the brainstem
    b. Loss of voluntary breathing control
    c. Damage to the cerebrum
    d. Toxicity of blood

MATCHING

Questions 22-27. Match the definition in column B to the correct term in column A.

Column A	Column B
22. _____ Medial	a. Toward the rear of the body
23. _____ Proximal	b. Toward midline
24. _____ Superior	c. Lying facedown
25. _____ Posterior	d. Movement away from the body
26. _____ Prone	
27. _____ Abduction	e. Toward the point of origin
	f. Toward the head

Questions 28-32. Match the type of spinal vertebrae in column A to the correct number found in the human spine in column B.

Column A	Column B
28. _____ Cervical vertebrae	a. Twelve mobile
29. _____ Thoracic vertebrae	b. Five fused
30. _____ Lumbar vertebrae	c. Seven mobile
31. _____ Sacrum	d. Four fused
32. _____ Coccyx	e. Five mobile

Questions 33-35. Match the type of muscle in column A to its function in column B.

Column A	Column B
33. _____ Voluntary or skeletal muscle	a. Movement of arms
34. _____ Involuntary or smooth muscle	b. Pumping of blood
35. _____ Cardiac muscle	c. Digestion

FILL IN THE BLANK

36. _____ is the anatomic term for "toward the front of the body."

37. _____ are vessels that direct blood flow away from the heart.

38. _____ is the anatomic term that means "on both sides."

39. _____ is the substance that connects the ribs to the sternum.

40. _____ is the layer of skin that houses the nerves.

41. The _____ is the respiratory muscle that separates the chest and abdomen.

42. Organs known as _____ filter liquid waste from the body.

43. _____ is another term for the "voice box."

44. _____ attaches bone to bone.

45. The _____ _____ is the large artery of the wrist and is used to check the pulse.

46. _____ attaches muscle to bone.

47. _____ is another term for the chest.

48. _____ is another term for the "windpipe."

49. _____ are vessels that direct blood flow toward the heart.

CASE SCENARIOS

Questions 50 to 53 refer to the following scenario.
You respond to a call at a construction site, where you find a 32-year-old woman who fell approximately 15 feet while working on the roof, landing on her right side. She is found lying on her back. As you evaluate the patient, you discover that she complains of pain to the back of her neck. You also find some swelling on the patient's left forearm, just below her elbow. The patient's left thigh is deformed approximately halfway between the hip and the knee. There is no break in the skin at the injury sites.
50. The position that you find the patient in is called:
    a. Prone
    b. Supine
    c. Trendelenburg
    d. Left lateral recumbent

51. When you make your radio presentation to the hospital, you describe the injury to the patient's forearm as:
    a. An injury to the humerus, proximal to the elbow
    b. An injury to the humerus, distal to the elbow
    c. An injury to the radius/ulna, superior to the elbow
    d. An injury to the radius/ulna, distal to the elbow
52. The injury to the thigh halfway between the hip and knee would best be described as:
    a. An injury to the proximal femur
    b. An injury to the midfemur
    c. An injury to the proximal humerus
    d. An injury to the midhumerus
53. After delivering the patient to the hospital, the physician compliments you on the way you treated this patient. The physician tells you that the x-ray film reveals that the patient sustained a fracture to her thoracic spine. You remember that the thoracic spine is composed of:
    a. Four vertebrae
    b. Five vertebrae
    c. Seven vertebrae
    d. Twelve vertebrae

Questions 54 to 57 refer to the following scenario.
You respond to a call for a 54-year-old man complaining of dizziness. During your evaluation the patient tells you that he was eating dinner when he began to choke on a piece of meat and could not breathe. His wife administered the Heimlich maneuver, which cleared the piece of meat, but the patient is now dizzy. When you further examine the patient, you notice that he has a very weak pulse and that his lips appear to be slightly blue in color.

54. You suspect that when the patient was choking, the piece of meat was lodged at or above this:
    a. Esophagus
    b. Vocal cords
    c. Bronchus
    d. Stomach

55. In documenting the patient's skin color on your prehospital care report, you would indicate that the patient appeared:
    a. Pale
    b. Flushed
    c. Jaundiced
    d. Cyanotic
56. Each beat of this patient's heart results in the pulse that you feel when you evaluate the patient. The pulse is generated when the:
    a. Atria contract
    b. Atria relax
    c. Ventricles contract
    d. Ventricles relax
57. The component of blood that when bound to oxygen gives skin its pink color and when *not* bound to oxygen gives skin a blue appearance is:
    a. White blood cells
    b. Plasma
    c. Platelets
    d. Hemoglobin

Question 58 refers to the following scenario.
You respond to an act of violence at a bar. As you approach the scene, you notice that it is safe and the police are on the scene. You are directed to evaluate a 23-year-old man who was punched in the left eye and kicked in the chest. The patient is found sitting at the curb and tells you that he is very upset. When you evaluate the patient, you determine that his pulse rate is 120 beats/min and that he is breathing rapidly.

58. As you continue your evaluation of this patient, you
    remember that the hormone _____ is released in times of stress.

19

59. Match the movement with the correct diagram in Fig. 4-1.

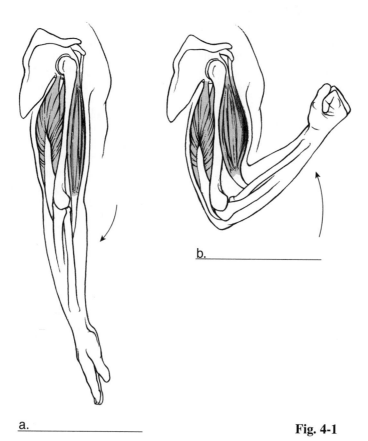

a. _____

b. _____

Fig. 4-1

Question	Choices
a. _____	Extension
b. _____	Flexion

60. Match the name of the bone with the correct location in Fig. 4-2.

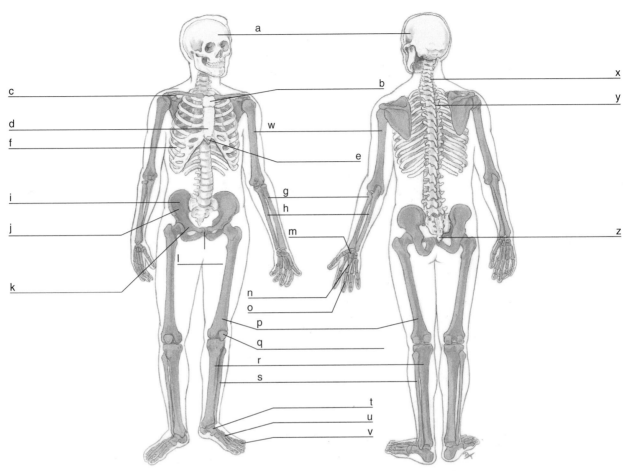

Fig. 4-2

<table>
<tr><td colspan="2" align="center">Question</td><td colspan="2" align="center">Choices</td></tr>
<tr><td>a. _____</td><td>n. _____</td><td>Carpals</td><td>Pelvis</td></tr>
<tr><td>b. _____</td><td>o. _____</td><td>Cervical vertebrae</td><td>Phalanges</td></tr>
<tr><td>c. _____</td><td>p. _____</td><td>Clavicle</td><td>Phalanges</td></tr>
<tr><td>d. _____</td><td>q. _____</td><td>Coccyx</td><td>Pubis</td></tr>
<tr><td>e. _____</td><td>r. _____</td><td>Femur</td><td>Radius</td></tr>
<tr><td>f. _____</td><td>s. _____</td><td>Fibula</td><td>Ribs</td></tr>
<tr><td>g. _____</td><td>t. _____</td><td>Humerus</td><td>Skull</td></tr>
<tr><td>h. _____</td><td>u. _____</td><td>Iliac crest</td><td>Sternum</td></tr>
<tr><td>i. _____</td><td>v. _____</td><td>Ischium</td><td>Tarsals</td></tr>
<tr><td>j. _____</td><td>w. _____</td><td>Manubrium</td><td>Thoracic vertebrae</td></tr>
<tr><td>k. _____</td><td>x. _____</td><td>Metacarpals</td><td>Tibia</td></tr>
<tr><td>l. _____</td><td>y. _____</td><td>Metatarsals</td><td>Ulna</td></tr>
<tr><td>m. _____</td><td>z. _____</td><td>Patella</td><td>Xiphoid process</td></tr>
</table>

Chapter **4 The Human Body**

61. Match the name of the bone with the correct location in Fig. 4-3.

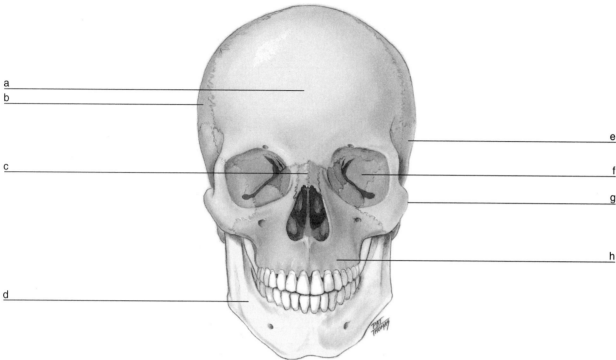

a
b

c

d

e

f

g

h

Fig. 4-3

Question

a. _____   e. _____
b. _____   f. _____
c. _____   g. _____
d. _____   h. _____

Choices

Frontal bone   Orbital bones
Mandible   Parietal bone
Maxilla   Temporal bone
Nasal bone   Zygomatic bone

62. Match the name of the structure with the correct location in Fig. 4-4.

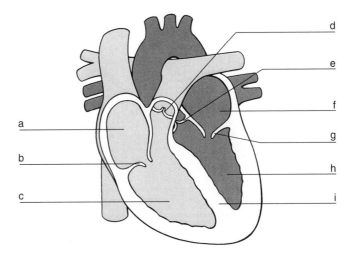

Fig. 4-4

Question		**Choices**	
a. _____	f. _____	Aortic valve	Right atrium
b. _____	g. _____	Left atrium	Right ventricle
c. _____	h. _____	Left ventricle	Tricuspid valve
d. _____	i. _____	Mitral valve	Ventricular septum
e. _____		Pulmonary valve	

63. Match the name of the structure with the correct location in Fig. 4-5.

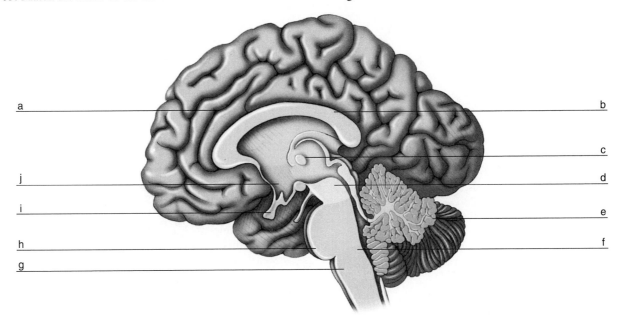

Fig. 4-5

Question		**Choices**	
a. _____	f. _____	Brainstem	Cerebrum
b. _____	g. _____	Midbrain	Medulla
c. _____	h. _____	Pituitary gland	Thalamus
d. _____	i. _____	Hypothalamus	Pons
e. _____	j. _____	Cerebellum	Corpus callosum

23

64. Match the name of the structure with the correct location in Fig. 4-6.

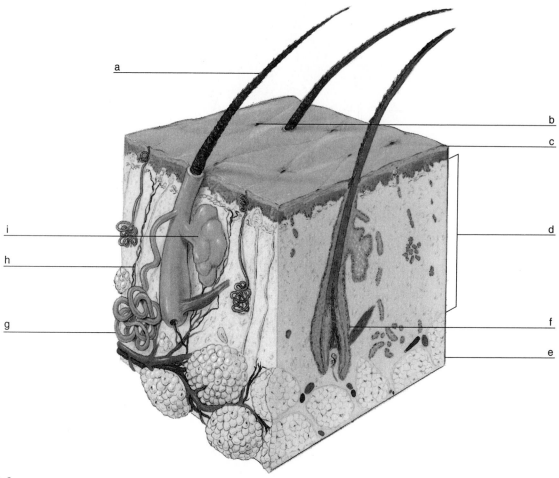

Fig. 4-6

Question		**Choices**	
a. _____	f. _____	Dermis	Nerve fiber
b. _____	g. _____	Sweat gland	Sweat pore
c. _____	h. _____	Hair shaft	Sebaceous (oil) gland
d. _____	i. _____	Hair follicle	Hypodermis
e. _____		Epidermis	

65. Match the name of the structure with the correct location in Fig. 4-7.

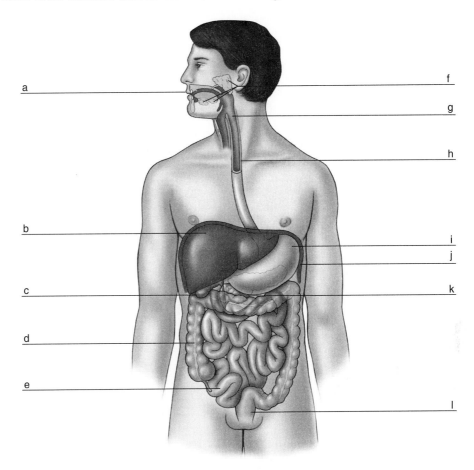

Fig. 4-7

<table>
<tr><th colspan="4">Question</th></tr>
<tr><td>a. _____</td><td>g. _____</td></tr>
<tr><td>b. _____</td><td>h. _____</td></tr>
<tr><td>c. _____</td><td>i. _____</td></tr>
<tr><td>d. _____</td><td>j. _____</td></tr>
<tr><td>e. _____</td><td>k. _____</td></tr>
<tr><td>f. _____</td><td>l. _____</td></tr>
</table>

Choices

Salivary glands	Mouth
Pharynx	Liver
Esophagus	Gallbladder
Diaphragm	Large intestine
Stomach	Small intestine
Pancreas	Rectum

66. Match the name of the structure with the correct location in Fig. 4-8.

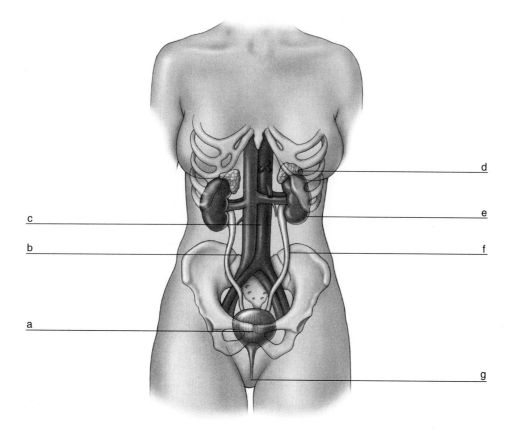

Fig. 4-8

Question		**Choices**	
a. _____	e. _____	Kidney	Abdominal aorta
b. _____	f. _____	Adrenal gland	Ureter
c. _____	g. _____	Urethra	Urinary bladder
d. _____		Common iliac vein	

Puzzle 4-1

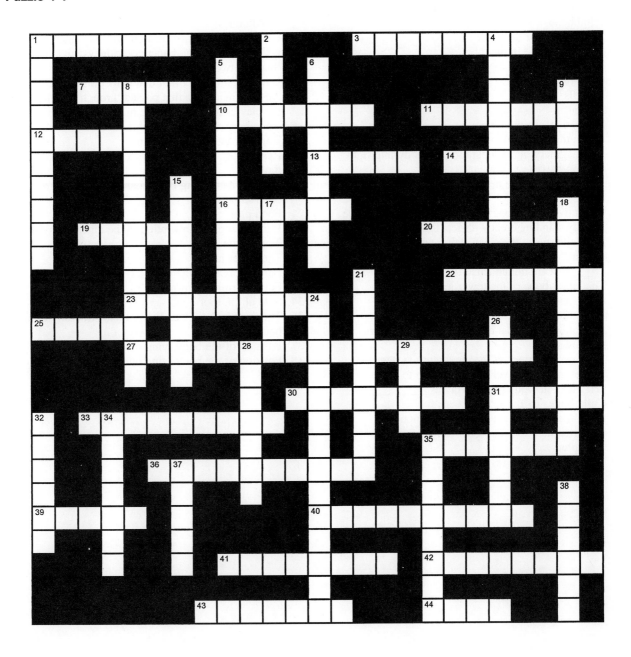

Chapter **4   The Human Body**

Across

1. Eight bones of the wrist
3. Large artery of the arm used in measuring blood pressure
7. Thighbone
10. Seven bones of the ankle
11. Artery palpable in the thigh
12. The fluid in which oxygen and nutrients are transported
13. Nostrils
14. Armpit
16. Bones that surround the eye
19. Organ that filters blood
20. An imaginary plane separating the body into right and left halves
22. Artery found in the neck used for pulse check
23. Navel
25. Collectively, the bones of the cranium and the face
27. A body standing erect with feet together and parallel, arms at the sides, palms and head facing forward
30. _____ ribs are not attached to the sternum
31. The larger bone of the lower leg
33. Outermost layer of skin
35. Breastbone
36. Flap of cartilage that covers the larynx during swallowing
39. The primary artery of the circulatory system
40. Nerve impulses travel from the brain to the peripheral nervous system via the _____ _____
41. Collarbone
42. Section of the spinal column that contains 12 vertebrae
43. Windpipe
44. The main organ of respiration

Down

1. Outpocketing of the brain located behind the brainstem
2. Section of the spinal column that contains five fused bones
4. Cavity that contains the stomach, intestines, liver, spleen, gallbladder, pancreas, kidneys, and ureters
5. Space between the ribs
6. Lower part of the brain that exits the skull
8. An imaginary line that passed through the middle of the clavicles parallel to the midline
9. Bone on the medial side of the forearm
15. Bones of the spinal column
17. Respiratory tubes that branch off just after the trachea
18. Protective covering that separates the heart from the other organs
21. Food pipe
24. Primary site for absorption in the digestive system
26. Toward the rear
28. The upper jaw
29. Largest organ of the body
32. Further from the trunk
34. Sole of the foot
35. The system that gives support and structure to the body
37. Position of the body lying on its face
38. Position of the body lying on its back

Puzzle 4-2

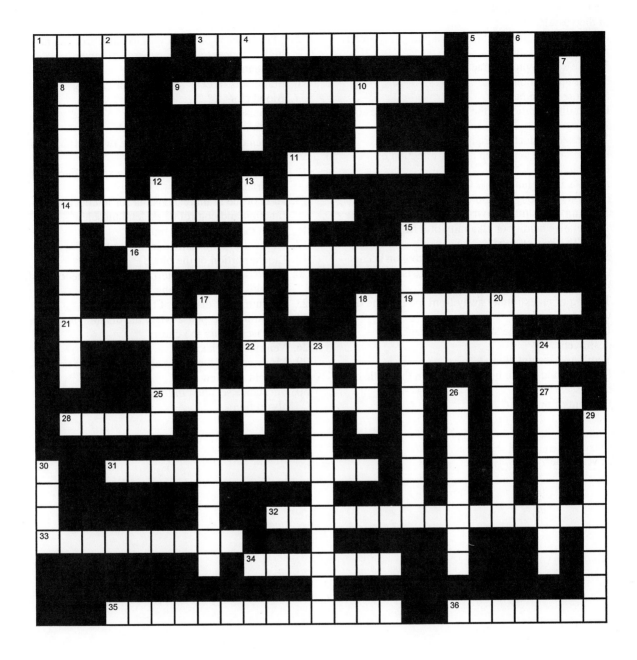

Across

1. Structures that maintain the one-way flow of blood in the vessels
3. Respiratory response when the diaphragm contracts and pushes downward
9. Muscle's ability to contract on its own
11. Sitting up position
14. Stopping of the heart
15. Bluish discoloration of the mucous membranes or skin
16. The waste product of respiration
19. Redness of the skin in an area of infection or inflammation
21. Air sacs in the lungs
22. Position of a body lying on its side
25. The sum of cellular activity
27. The relative acidity or alkalinity of a fluid
28. Partially digested food
31. Membrane that is surgically opened to gain access to the airway when an obstruction exists above the larynx
32. Turning of an extremity away from the midline of the body
33. Disease in which the alveoli are damaged or destroyed
34. Ventricular contraction
35. Force exerted by the blood volume on the walls of the vessels
36. Pigment of the skin

Down

2. _____ muscles are controlled by a person's will
4. Hypoperfusion
5. The tendency of molecules to move from an area of higher concentration to an area of lower concentration
6. Fragments of cells necessary for clotting
7. Blood clot
8. No pulse and no respirations
10. Fundamental unit of all living things
11. Movement of a joint so that the two parts are closer together
12. The amount of air inspired and expired during one respiratory cycle
13. Area of the brain responsible for intellectual function and control of skeletal muscles
15. Fluid that protects the brain
17. Amount of air breathed in 1 minute
18. Liquid portion of the blood
20. Blood disorder characterized by a deficiency of the proteins used for clotting
23. Inflammatory disease of the epiglottis
24. Respiratory response when the diaphragm relaxes and rises within the chest
26. Ventricular relaxation
29. Movement of the elbow from the bent to the straight position
30. Substance secreted in the liver that aids fat absorption

5 Lifting and Moving Patients

MULTIPLE CHOICE

1. The scientific method of efficiently lifting large weights so as *not* to injure oneself is best described as:
   a. Ergonomics
   b. Body mechanics
   c. Body preservation
   d. Longevity
2. When lifting a patient, you should use the muscles in your:
   a. Lower back
   b. Upper back
   c. Legs
   d. Pelvis
3. When carrying a stretcher with a patient on it, your back should be:
   a. Flexed
   b. Hyperextended
   c. Held straight
   d. Curved
4. When performing a patient lift, your arms should be:
   a. As close to your body as possible
   b. As far apart as possible
   c. Flexed at the elbow
   d. With palms facing downward
5. A one-handed carry with a stretcher can be used when:
   a. There are only two people available for the carry.
   b. You need to compensate for an imbalance.
   c. There are multiple people available for the carry.
   d. You cannot maintain a straight posture.
6. When using the one-handed carry technique, the EMT should:
   a. Keep the back in a locked position.
   b. Keep the back in the flexed position.
   c. Compensate for the imbalance.
   d. Flex at the waist when picking up the object with one hand.
7. Which of the following statements is correct when carrying a patient down a flight of stairs?
   a. The EMT at the bottom of the device will have most of the weight.
   b. The EMT at the top of the device will have most of the weight.
   c. Each EMT shares the weight distribution equally.
   d. The incline has no bearing on the distribution of the weight.
8. Back injuries to the EMT typically occur:
   a. When using the one-handed carry.
   b. When carrying a patient down the stairs.
   c. When reaching or stretching during the lifting process.
   d. When lifting a patient into the ambulance.

9. When reaching or stretching, the EMT should reach no more than:
   a. 5 to 10 inches from the body
   b. 15 to 20 inches from the body
   c. 20 to 25 inches from the body
   d. 30 to 35 inches from the body
10. When performing a log roll, the EMT positioned at the patient's _____ should supervise the movements.
    a. head
    b. shoulder
    c. hip
    d. lower leg
11. Before performing a log roll on a patient who fell 30 feet, the EMT should:
    a. Tie the patient's hands and legs together.
    b. Immobilize the cervical spine.
    c. Obtain written consent.
    d. Ask if the patient can move the head from side to side.
12. When pushing or pulling a patient to the ambulance, it is important to:
    a. Pull, because it is safer than pushing.
    b. Push, because it is safer than pulling.
    c. Carry the patient whenever possible, because it is more stable than pushing or pulling.
    d. Keep elbows locked while pushing or pulling.
13. The method for quickly removing a patient in respiratory arrest from a car is called:
    a. Load and go
    b. Rapid extrication
    c. Scoop and run
    d. Triage

FILL IN THE BLANK

14. Patients in the late stages of pregnancy should be transported in the _____ _____ _____ position.

15. The simplest technique for moving a patient who is in immediate danger from a fire or an explosion is the _____ _____.

16. The primary concern for unconscious patients is _____ management.

MATCHING

Questions 17-23. Match the device in column A with its primary use in column B.

Column A

17. _____ Wheeled cot
18. _____ Stair chair
19. _____ Vest-type device
20. _____ Long spine board
21. _____ Scoop stretcher
22. _____ Stokes basket
23. _____ Flexible (Reeve's) stretcher

Column B: Primary Use of Device

a. Used to move patients over rough terrain or during high-angle rescues.
b. The primary device for immobilizing the supine patient.
c. Aluminum device that splits lengthwise to facilitate moving the patient off the ground.
d. The primary device to move the conscious medical patient up or down stairs.
e. Used for carrying a patient through narrow corridors.
f. The preferred device for transporting a patient along smooth terrain.
g. Used to immobilize and extricate the seated patient from an automobile.

CASE SCENARIOS

Questions 24 to 26 refer to the following scenario.
You respond to a motor vehicle incident and find a woman walking around outside the car. She informs you that she was driving the car when it was hit in the rear by another car. Another EMS crew is caring for the patient in the second car. Your patient is complaining of neck pain.

24. The best device that you can use to immobilize this patient is a:
    a. Long spine board
    b. Stokes basket
    c. Scoop stretcher
    d. Vest-type device

25. As you immobilize this patient to the appropriate device, you use:
    a. A cervical collar with a head immobilization device; the torso and legs do not need to be secured to the device.
    b. A cervical collar with a head immobilization device, securing the torso and the legs to the device.
    c. Straps to secure the head, torso, and legs to the device; a cervical collar is not needed once the patient is on the device.
    d. A head immobilization device along with straps to secure the torso and legs to the device.

26. You notice that the second EMS crew is caring for their patient, who is lying supine on the pavement. You would expect the EMS crew to move the patient by:
    a. Using an extremity carry and placing the patient on a long spine board.
    b. Using an extremity carry and placing the patient directly on the ambulance stretcher.
    c. Using the log roll to place the patient on a long spine board.
    d. Using the vest-type device to move the patient to the ambulance stretcher.

Questions 27 and 28 refer to the following scenario.
You respond to a call and find a 43-year-old man on the second floor of a house complaining of abdominal pain. The patient tells you that he has a history of gallbladder disease and he thinks he is having another gallbladder attack. Because of the pain the patient tells you that he cannot walk down the stairs.

27. The best device to move this patient down the stairs is the:
    a. Ambulance stretcher
    b. Long spine board
    c. Scoop stretcher
    d. Stair chair

28. The position of comfort for most patients complaining of abdominal pain is:
    a. Supine
    b. Prone
    c. Supine with the knees bent
    d. Supine with the head elevated

29. Put the following steps for rapid extrication in proper sequential order.

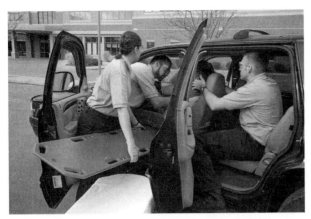

a. A third EMT prepares the stretcher and places the backboard under the patient's leg.

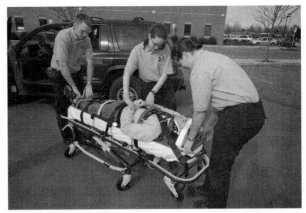

d. After being moved out of the vehicle and onto the stretcher, the patient is strapped to the backboard and then secured to the stretcher.

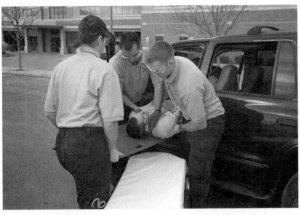

b. The patient is placed flat on the backboard. Maintaining control of the patient's head and neck, the EMTs slide the patient onto the backboard.

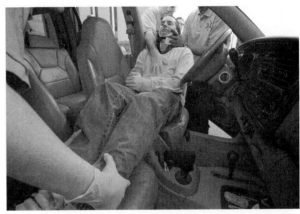

e. In unison, the second EMT takes control of the patient's neck as the first EMT moves to rotate the patient onto the backboard. A fourth EMT positioned next to the patient in the vehicle moves the patient's legs across the seat.

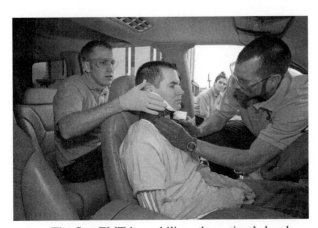

c. The first EMT immobilizes the patient's head from the back. The second EMT sizes and places a neck collar.

Correct Order

1. _____

2. _____

3. _____

4. _____

5. _____

33

6 Airway

MULTIPLE CHOICE

1. The structure that covers the trachea during swallowing to prevent aspiration is called the:
   a. Pharynx
   b. Epiglottis
   c. Thyroid cartilage
   d. Cricoid cartilage

2. The respiratory structure that is palpable just above the sternum is the:
   a. Bronchus
   b. Trachea
   c. Carina
   d. Bronchiole

3. The muscle that separates the chest and abdomen is called the:
   a. Diaphragm
   b. Intercostal
   c. Abdominis recti
   d. None of the above

4. The normal resting tidal volume for an adult is approximately:
   a. 500 mL
   b. 800 mL
   c. 1000 mL
   d. 2000 mL

5. The process by which gases move from an area of higher concentration to an area of lower concentration is called:
   a. Ventilation
   b. Respiration
   c. Diffusion
   d. Transportation

6. The portion of the lung where diffusion takes place is called the:
   a. Bronchi
   b. Pleura
   c. Bronchiole
   d. Alveoli

7. When the brainstem sends messages to the intercostals and diaphragm, they contract and increase the size of the thoracic cavity. At that point, the pressure within the thoracic cavity:
   a. Increases
   b. Decreases
   c. Remains the same
   d. None of the above

8. The amount of air inhaled and exhaled during a given breath is called the:
   a. Residual volume
   b. Expiratory reserve
   c. Total volume
   d. Tidal volume

9. What percentage of oxygen does normal atmospheric air contain?
   a. 15%
   b. 21%
   c. 28%
   d. 50%

10. The portion of the brain responsible for regulation of breathing is called the:
    a. Cerebrum
    b. Cerebellum
    c. Hypothalamus
    d. Brainstem

11. During positive-pressure ventilation, adequate tidal volume is evaluated primarily on the basis of:
    a. Chest rise
    b. Skin color
    c. Pupil response
    d. None of the above

12. The most common complication of excessive or forceful ventilation is:
    a. Pneumothorax
    b. Gastric distention
    c. Oxygen toxicity
    d. Air embolism

13. Which of the following administration devices results in the highest oxygen delivery to the patient?
    a. Nasal cannula
    b. Venturi mask
    c. Nonrebreather mask
    d. Simple face mask

14. The most common cause of airway obstruction is:
    a. Allergic reactions
    b. Food
    c. The tongue
    d. Trauma to the airway

15. In patients with suspected spinal trauma, the manual airway maneuver of choice is the:
    a. Jaw thrust without head tilt
    b. Head-tilt/neck-lift
    c. Head-tilt/chin-lift
    d. Tongue pull

16. The correct ventilation rate for a nonbreathing adult patient is one breath every:
    a. 3 seconds
    b. 4 seconds
    c. 5 seconds
    d. 6 seconds

17. In the absence of spinal injury, the airway maneuver of choice is the:
    a. Modified jaw thrust
    b. Head-tilt/neck-lift
    c. Head-tilt/chin-lift
    d. Tongue pull

35

18. When inserting an oropharyngeal airway, the patient begins to gag and choke. Your next action should be to:
    a. Remove the airway.
    b. Use a smaller airway.
    c. Lubricate the airway.
    d. Tape the airway in place.
19. To ensure proper sizing, an oropharyngeal airway is measured from the corner of the patient's mouth to the:
    a. Angle of the jaw
    b. Top of the ear
    c. Cheekbone
    d. Trachea
20. The pocket mask used in conjunction with 15 L of oxygen per minute can result in maximum oxygen concentrations of approximately:
    a. 16%
    b. 21%
    c. 30%
    d. 50%
21. The major complication of a bag-mask resuscitator is:
    a. Overventilation and pneumothorax
    b. Low tidal volumes caused by errors in technique
    c. Rupture of the bag during exhalation
    d. Valve failure from clogging
22. What is the maximum percentage of oxygen delivery for a bag-mask used with an oxygen reservoir?
    a. 25% to 35%
    b. 50% to 60%
    c. 75% to 80%
    d. 90% to 100%
23. To avoid confusion with other gases, an oxygen tank is painted:
    a. Blue
    b. Purple
    c. Red
    d. Green
24. The tank pressure of a full oxygen cylinder is usually (psi, pounds per square inch):
    a. 700 psi
    b. 1000 psi
    c. 2000 psi
    d. 4000 psi
25. The system used to avoid misplacement of a regulator on portable oxygen cylinders is called the:
    a. Oxygen cylinder safety system
    b. Pin index safety system
    c. Gas delivery safety system
    d. Regulator safety system
26. Which of the following oxygen cylinders is the most portable?
    a. D cylinder
    b. G cylinder
    c. H cylinder
    d. M cylinder

27. Regulators are designed to provide a safe pressure to the delivery device of approximately:
    a. 10 to 20 psi
    b. 20 to 30 psi
    c. 40 to 70 psi
    d. 100 to 120 psi
28. A flowmeter that uses a gravity-controlled ball to measure the liter flow rates to the delivery device is called a:
    a. Bourdon gauge
    b. Pressure-compensated flowmeter
    c. Constant-flow selector
    d. Double-staged flowmeter
29. When suctioning the upper airway, you should activate the negative pressure:
    a. When the tip is in the oropharynx
    b. Before insertion
    c. At the entrance of the mouth
    d. Halfway between the teeth and the pharynx
30. Lifting at the angles of the jaw while maintaining the head in the neutral inline position best describes the:
    a. Modified jaw thrust
    b. Head-tilt/chin-lift
    c. Chin pull
    d. Tongue-jaw lift
31. The best way to remove liquid secretions from the airway in the field is by:
    a. Finger sweeps
    b. Back blows
    c. Portable suction
    d. Abdominal thrusts
32. When using a jaw thrust in conjunction with bag-mask device, you can lift the mandible at the:
    a. Center of the chin
    b. Angle of the jaw
    c. Lower portion of the cheekbones
    d. Soft tissues of the mandible
33. When using the bag-mask, the major advantage of two rescuers is that this method:
    a. Decreases leakage of air from a two-handed mask seal.
    b. Decreases fatigue of the rescuers involved in the resuscitation.
    c. Ensures a smoother bag squeeze during the breath.
    d. Positions the rescuers at the head of the patient.
34. To ensure proper delivery of volume when using a flow-restricted, oxygen-powered ventilation device, you should release the lever (or button) when:
    a. A whistling sound occurs.
    b. You observe adequate chest rise.
    c. Resistance is encountered.
    d. The cheeks are distended.
35. To ensure proper sizing, a nasopharyngeal airway is measured from the tip of the nose to the:
    a. Angle of the jaw
    b. Middle of the ear
    c. Cheekbone
    d. Larynx

36. When a patient cannot tolerate a nonrebreather mask, you should:
   a. Place it over the nose or corner of the mouth.
   b. Switch to a nasal cannula.
   c. Hold the mask firmly in place.
   d. Lay the patient supine to decrease anxiety.

MATCHING

Questions 37 and 38. Match the delivery device in column B to the appropriate oxygen concentrations in column A.

Column A	Column B
37. 90% at 10 to 15 L	a. Nasal cannula
38. 24% to 40% at 2 to 6 L	b. Nonrebreather mask

FILL IN THE BLANK

39. The tidal volume multiplied by the respiratory rate is called the _____ _____.

40. The nose is divided into two compartments by the _____ _____.

41. Blue-gray skin color is called _____.

42. Low oxygen content in the blood is called _____.

43. When delivering positive-pressure ventilation, _____ _____ can be used to compress the esophagus, thereby reducing the chances of gastric distention.

44. The narrowest part of the pediatric airway is at the ring formed by the _____ _____.

CASE SCENARIOS

Questions 45 to 49 refer to the following scenario.
You respond to a call at a shopping center and encounter an approximately 3-year-old boy who is having a seizure. Bystanders tell you that the patient has been seizing for the past 5 minutes. The patient exhibits signs of seizure activity; his teeth are clenched closed, and his lips appear to be blue.

45. The best way to establish an airway in this patient is to:
   a. Force the patient's teeth apart and insert an oropharyngeal airway.
   b. Insert a nasopharyngeal airway.
   c. There is no need to establish an airway; wait until seizure activity stops, and then assess the patient's respiratory status.
   d. Apply a nasal cannula at 2 L/min.

46. The procedures needed to insert an airway device in this patient require that:
   a. The bevel is facing toward the septum.
   b. The bevel is facing away from the septum.
   c. Whatever pressure is needed to insert the device is used.
   d. Another airway device is used if the airway cannot be inserted successfully in one nostril.

47. Once the child's seizure activity stops, you determine that the patient is *not* breathing. The best device to use to ventilate this patient is:
   a. Mouth-to-mouth ventilations
   b. A bag-mask device without supplemental oxygen
   c. A flow-restricted, oxygen-powered ventilator
   d. A bag-mask device connected to 15 L/min of oxygen

48. The volume of air that you use to ventilate this patient with each breath is called the:
   a. Minute volume
   b. Residual volume
   c. Tidal volume
   d. Stroke volume

49. The rate at which you will ventilate this patient is:
   a. 8 to 10 times per minute
   b. 10 to 12 times per minute
   c. 10 to 15 times per minute
   d. 12 to 20 times per minute

Questions 50 to 53 refer to the following scenario.
You respond to a call from a restaurant, where you find a 67-year-old woman unconscious and unresponsive on the floor. The patient has a pulse but is not breathing. When you evaluate the patient's airway, you notice large quantities of partially chewed food in the patient's mouth.

50. The best way to clear this patient's airway is to:
   a. Insert an oropharyngeal airway.
   b. Insert a nasopharyngeal airway.
   c. Use your gloved fingers to sweep out as much debris as possible.
   d. Use a suction device with a soft catheter.

51. After you clear the patient's airway, you begin to provide positive-pressure ventilations. The rate at which you will ventilate this patient is:
   a. 8 to 10 times per minute
   b. 10 to 12 times per minute
   c. 10 to 15 times per minute
   d. 12 to 20 times per minute

52. En route to the hospital the patient begins to vomit, resulting in large quantities of liquid vomitus in the patient's mouth. You should:
   a. Suction continuously until you arrive at the hospital.
   b. Use the suction device for no more than 15 seconds.
   c. Insert an oropharyngeal airway, which will allow for uninterrupted ventilations.
   d. Use a flow-restricted, oxygen-powered ventilator to clear the airway.

53. While you provide positive-pressure ventilation to your patient, you instruct your partner to apply downward pressure to the patient's neck in an effort to close the esophagus and reduce the amount of air entering the patient's stomach. This is called:
    a. Cricoid pressure
    b. Tracheal pressure
    c. Esophageal pressure
    d. Tracheal deviation

Questions 54 to 58 refer to the following scenario.
You respond to a call for a patient who was struck by a car. The scene has been secured by the police and fire department before your arrival. You find a 42-year-old man lying on his face in the roadway. The patient does not respond to verbal or painful stimuli.

54. The position that you find this patient in is called:
    a. Supine
    b. Trendelenburg
    c. Prone
    d. Left lateral recumbent

55. Your first steps in treating this patient include:
    a. Immobilizing the patient in the position you find him and transporting him rapidly to the hospital.
    b. Performing a log roll to position the patient on his back while maintaining cervical spinal immobilization.
    c. Placing the patient in the left lateral recumbent position to maintain an open airway.
    d. Applying nasal cannula oxygen to the patient while you begin to immobilize him in the position that you found him.

56. Once you have properly immobilized the patient, you open his airway by using:
    a. The head-tilt/chin-lift method
    b. The head-tilt/jaw-lift maneuver
    c. The jaw thrust maneuver
    d. A blanket roll under the patient's neck

57. You begin to transport your patient to the hospital. You are alone with the patient in the back of the ambulance when the patient stops breathing. The best way for you, as a single rescuer, to ventilate this patient is by:
    a. Performing mouth-to-mouth ventilations.
    b. Performing a head tilt to open the airway while ventilating with a bag-mask device.
    c. Performing a jaw thrust to open the airway while ventilating with a pocket mask.
    d. Using a nonrebreather oxygen mask.

58. On arrival at the hospital, you continue to support your patient's respirations while providing supplemental oxygen. Your portable oxygen tank, which you bring with you into the hospital, is a:
    a. D cylinder
    b. G cylinder
    c. H cylinder
    d. M cylinder

59. Put the following steps in the emergency treatment of adult choking in proper sequential order.

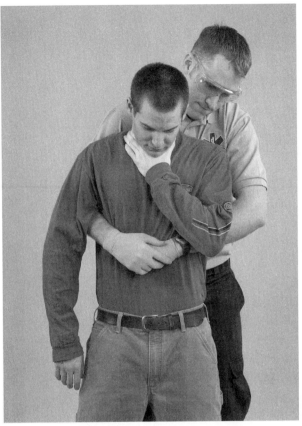

a. Give abdominal thrusts. (Use chest thrusts for pregnant or obese victims.) Repeat thrusts until object is expelled or the victim becomes unresponsive.

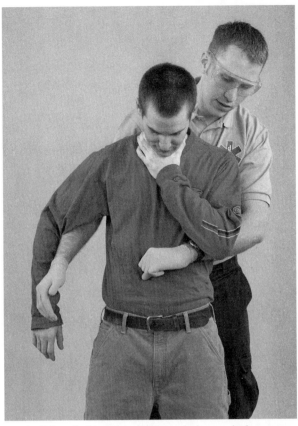

b. Move behind the choking victim, and place one hand on the person's abdomen above the umbilicus and below the ribs. Reach around the victim with your other hand and grab the first hand, holding firmly.

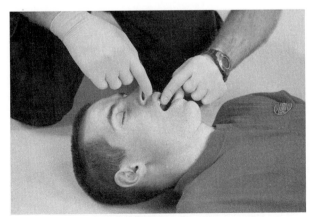

c. If the victim becomes unresponsive, help the person safely to the ground. Perform a tongue-jaw lift followed by a finger sweep to remove the object if you see it.

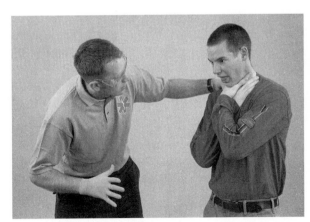

d. Ask, "Are you choking?"

39

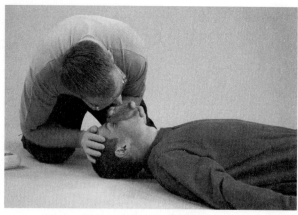

e. Attempt to ventilate the patient.

f. If unable to ventilate, begin CPR. Every time you attempt a breath, look for the object and remove it if you see it.

Correct Order

1. _____
2. _____
3. _____
4. _____
5. _____
6. _____
7. _____

7 Patient Assessment

MULTIPLE CHOICE

1. The best method for evaluating the adequacy of ventilation is by:
   a. Observing chest rise.
   b. Placing a mirror near the mouth and nose.
   c. Feeling the chest wall for expansion.
   d. Checking the pulse rate.
2. The correct location of palpation for the carotid pulse is:
   a. At the groove between the larynx and muscle in the neck.
   b. At the angle of the jaw adjacent to the muscle.
   c. Just above the suprasternal notch.
   d. Just above the clavicle, adjacent to the trachea.
3. The carotid pulse should be palpated on:
   a. Either side of the neck.
   b. The side opposite the rescuer.
   c. The same side as the rescuer.
   d. Both sides of the neck each time.
4. Which of the following questions reflects the best way to inquire about a chest pain complaint in a medical history?
   a. Was your chest pain squeezing in nature?
   b. How would you describe the pain in your own words?
   c. Did it feel like someone was standing on your chest?
   d. Was the pain viselike in nature?
5. The expression of the patient's main complaint in his or her own words is called the:
   a. History of present illness
   b. Primary problem
   c. Primary complaint
   d. Chief complaint
6. The normal range of respiratory rate in the adult is approximately _____ breaths/min.
   a. 5 to 15
   b. 10 to 15
   c. 12 to 20
   d. 15 to 25
7. The artery routinely used to monitor the pulse in the conscious adult patient is the:
   a. Radial
   b. Femoral
   c. Brachial
   d. Ulnar
8. The normal range of pulse rate for an adult at rest is approximately _____ beats/min.
   a. 40 to 60
   b. 50 to 70
   c. 60 to 80
   d. 80 to 120
9. The diastolic blood pressure is recorded on the basis of when:
   a. Auscultated sounds diminish or disappear.
   b. Auscultated sounds first appear.
   c. Palpated pulses disappear.
   d. Palpated pulses are first felt.
10. Blood pressure determined by listening through a stethoscope is called blood pressure by:
    a. Auscultation
    b. Palpation
    c. Oscillation
    d. Vibration
11. Which artery is routinely monitored while auscultating a blood pressure?
    a. Radial
    b. Brachial
    c. Ulnar
    d. Femoral
12. What is the component of blood pressure associated with the first sound heard through the stethoscope?
    a. Diastolic
    b. Systolic
    c. Pulse
    d. Contractile
13. Which component of blood pressure is obtained when using the palpation technique?
    a. Diastolic
    b. Systolic
    c. Pulse
    d. Contractile
14. The pulse that can be palpated in the anterolateral aspect of the wrist, just below the thumb, is the:
    a. Brachial
    b. Ulnar
    c. Radial
    d. Humeral
15. What is the main reason why baseline vital signs are so important to the care of the patient?
    a. Patients expect their vital signs to be taken and would be suspicious of care if you did not take them.
    b. Vital signs provide a baseline value by which the effectiveness of therapy can be measured.
    c. To prevent legal problems related to the care of the patient if you are sued at a later time.
    d. To compare one patient with another for quality assurance studies related to vital sign changes.

16. What is the pulse of a patient in severe shock likely to feel like?
    a. Strong and slow
    b. Weak and rapid
    c. Strong and irregular
    d. Weak and irregular
17. Capillary refill in a child is considered delayed when the refilling time is:
    a. Less than 1 second
    b. 1 second
    c. 2 seconds
    d. Greater than 2 seconds
18. Which of the following skin colors is associated with impaired blood flow and poor perfusion?
    a. Pale
    b. Flushed
    c. Jaundiced
    d. Cherry red
19. Which skin color is often associated with abnormalities with the liver?
    a. Cyanotic
    b. Pale
    c. Flushed
    d. Jaundiced
20. Which of the following descriptions best describes normal pupils?
    a. Midpositional, equal, and reactive
    b. Dilated, equal, and reactive
    c. Constricted, equal, and nonreactive
    d. Dilated, equal, and nonreactive
21. Which of the following pupils would you describe as "normally reactive"?
    a. A pupil that becomes larger when a light is projected into the eye.
    b. A pupil that becomes smaller when a light is projected into the eye.
    c. A pupil that is unchanged when a light is projected into the eye.
    d. A pupil that becomes larger, then smaller when a light is projected into the eye.
22. What is the skin assessment of a patient in shock likely to reveal?
    a. Cool, moist skin
    b. Warm, moist skin
    c. Cool, dry skin
    d. Warm, dry skin
23. Which of the following is a *sign*?
    a. Chest pain
    b. Nausea
    c. Swollen ankles
    d. Dizziness
24. Gathering information from bystanders, identifying hazards, securing the scene, and calling for specialized assistance are all components of the:
    a. Focused (secondary) assessment
    b. Scene size-up
    c. Secondary survey
    d. Dispatch review

25. Which of the following pupils is most constricted?

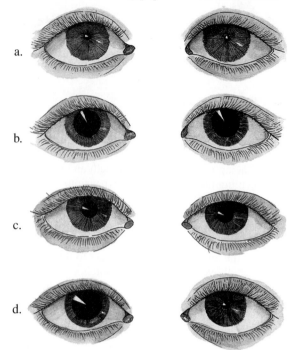

a.

b.

c.

d.

26. The routine practice of wearing protective clothing (e.g., gloves, goggles) when performing certain procedures (e.g., bleeding control) is called:
    a. General infection prevention
    b. Barrier protection model
    c. Immunization techniques
    d. Standard precautions
27. When splash from a bleeding artery is possible, the recommended personal protective equipment includes:
    a. Mask, goggles, gown, and gloves
    b. Mask only
    c. Gloves only
    d. Gown and goggles only
28. When delivering a baby, the recommended personal protective equipment is the wearing of:
    a. Mask, goggles, gown, and gloves
    b. Mask only
    c. Gloves only
    d. Gown and goggles only
29. When bandaging a minor abrasion where splash of blood is *not* likely, the recommended personal protective equipment is the wearing of:
    a. Mask, goggles, and gown
    b. Mask only
    c. Gloves only
    d. Gown and goggles only

30. A good rule of thumb for approaching a potentially hazardous scene is to stop and evaluate from a position:
    a. 100 feet away, uphill, and upwind
    b. 50 feet away, downhill, and downwind
    c. 100 feet away, downhill, and downwind
    d. 50 feet away, uphill, and upwind
31. Using the rule of thumb for placing traffic delineation devices on a highway, what is the minimum distance they should be placed from an incident on a 50-mph road?
    a. 50 feet
    b. 100 feet
    c. 150 feet
    d. 200 feet
32. After ensuring that the scene is safe, it is important to identify the mechanism of injury and determine the total number of patients at the scene so that the:
    a. Initial (primary) assessment is more organized.
    b. Need for additional resources is identified.
    c. Workload can be distributed between you and your partner.
    d. Appropriate lifting equipment can be secured.
33. You arrive at a scene where there are 12 injured patients. After ensuring scene safety, what should you do first?
    a. Call for additional units.
    b. Begin triage.
    c. Begin your initial (primary) assessment.
    d. Begin treating the most serious patients.
34. The process of identifying the underlying cause of an illness or injury is called identifying the:
    a. Initial pathology
    b. Detailed assessment finding
    c. Focused physical cause
    d. Mechanism of injury or illness
35. The general impression is a series of initial questions and observations regarding the patient's condition, age, gender, and chief complaint and is designed to identify:
    a. Scene safety
    b. Life-threatening conditions
    c. A diagnosis
    d. Underlying pathophysiology
36. After establishing unresponsiveness in a prone trauma patient, you should:
    a. Leave the patient in the prone position and continue with your survey.
    b. Log-roll the patient to the lateral recumbent position and continue with your survey.
    c. Log-roll the patient to the supine position and continue with your survey.
    d. Leave the patient in the prone position and transport immediately.

37. The V of the AVPU evaluation of mental state refers to a patient's ability to respond to:
    a. Vigorous stimuli
    b. Verbal stimuli
    c. Visual stimuli
    d. Vivid stimuli
38. When opening the airway of an infant to assess breathing, you should place the head in the:
    a. Neutral or sniffing position
    b. Hyperextended position
    c. Slightly flexed position
    d. Elevated position
39. Tilting the head back with one hand while lifting the lower margin of the jaw with the index and middle fingers of the other hand best describes the:
    a. Jaw thrust without head tilt
    b. Chin pull maneuver
    c. Head-tilt/neck-lift
    d. Head-tilt/chin-lift
40. The best method for evaluating the adequacy of ventilation is by:
    a. Observing chest rise.
    b. Placing a mirror near the mouth and nose.
    c. Feeling the chest wall for expansion.
    d. Checking the pulse rate.
41. The correct location of palpation for the carotid pulse is:
    a. A groove between the larynx and muscle in the neck.
    b. At the angle of the jaw adjacent to the muscle.
    c. Just above the suprasternal notch.
    d. Just above the clavicle, adjacent to the trachea.
42. In general, the carotid pulse should be palpated on:
    a. Either side of the neck.
    b. The side opposite the EMT.
    c. The same side as the EMT.
    d. Both sides of the neck each time.
43. The carotid pulse should be initially palpated for approximately:
    a. 2 to 3 seconds
    b. 3 to 5 seconds
    c. 5 to 10 seconds
    d. 10 to 20 seconds
44. Capillary refill in the child is considered delayed when refill takes more than:
    a. 0.5 second
    b. 1 second
    c. 1.5 seconds
    d. 2 seconds
45. Inline immobilization of the cervical spine is essential in trauma patients to avoid injury to the:
    a. Brain
    b. Soft tissues of the neck
    c. Bony structures
    d. Spinal cord

46. When a patient has adequate breathing but is short of breath, he or she should be treated with:
    a. Oxygen
    b. A bag-mask
    c. Psychological care only
    d. A flow-restricted, oxygen-powered ventilation device

47. A patient who is unresponsive and breathing at a rate of 5 breaths/min should be treated with:
    a. Nonrebreather mask
    b. Bag-mask with supplemental oxygen
    c. Psychological care only
    d. Venturi mask

48. Which of the following signs is common to infants and small children but *not* adults?
    a. Nasal flaring
    b. Accessory muscle use
    c. Cyanosis
    d. Decreased breath sounds

49. A 6-month-old infant's pulse should initially be palpated at which artery?
    a. Carotid
    b. Radial
    c. Femoral
    d. Brachial

50. Which of the following would be checked during the initial (primary) assessment?
    a. Contusions on the head
    b. External bleeding
    c. Instability of the pelvic bone
    d. Abdominal distention

51. Skin color that is cyanotic usually reflects:
    a. Poorly oxygenated red blood cells
    b. Hypothermia of tissues
    c. Hyperthermia
    d. Liver disease

52. Which of the following skin findings are usually associated with shock states?
    a. Pale, cool, and clammy
    b. Flushed, warm, and dry
    c. Cyanotic, warm, and dry
    d. Jaundiced, cool, and dry

53. Which of the following skin findings is most likely in a patient with complete airway obstruction?
    a. Pale
    b. Flushed
    c. Cyanotic
    d. Jaundiced

54. Which of the following statements best explains the reason for performing a rapid trauma assessment?
    a. Internal bleeding must be identified early and controlled at the scene.
    b. EMT medications may be lifesaving for serious head injuries.
    c. To avoid prolonged discomfort to the patient associated with the examination.
    d. To identify serious conditions that might not be identified by the initial (primary) assessment alone.

55. Signs and symptoms, allergies, medications, past medical history, last meal, and events leading up to the problem are components of a:
    a. General impression
    b. Past medical history
    c. SAMPLE history
    d. Chief complaint

56. The three major diseases that are routinely inquired about during the past medical history in older adult patients are:
    a. Heart disease, chronic pulmonary disease, high blood pressure
    b. Heart disease, diabetes, HIV infection
    c. Diabetes, chronic pulmonary disease, high blood pressure
    d. Heart disease, diabetes, high blood pressure

57. How many breaths per minute is the normal range of respiratory rate for the adult patient?
    a. 5 to 15
    b. 10 to 15
    c. 12 to 20
    d. 15 to 25

58. The artery routinely used to monitor the rate, regularity, and quality of the pulse in the conscious adult patient is the:
    a. Radial
    b. Femoral
    c. Brachial
    d. Ulnar

59. Blood pressure determined by listening through a stethoscope is called blood pressure by:
    a. Auscultation
    b. Palpation
    c. Oscillation
    d. Vibration

60. The muscles used to determine the presence of respiratory distress are called the:
    a. Deltoid muscles
    b. Pectoral muscles
    c. Diaphragm muscles
    d. Accessory muscles

61. Air beneath the skin that is characterized by a crackling sensation during palpation of the neck and upper chest is called:
    a. Coarse rales
    b. Dermatitis pneumonia
    c. Subcutaneous emphysema
    d. Crepitant rales

62. The structure that can be palpated midline above the sternum is called the:
    a. Esophagus
    b. Pharynx
    c. Glottis
    d. Trachea

63. The rapid trauma assessment is designed to search for:
    a. All possible injuries to the patient
    b. Injuries in the head and trunk area
    c. Injuries that are minor
    d. Life-threatening injuries

64. Breath sounds should routinely be auscultated on the upper anterior chest (apices) and:
    a. Laterally at the bases
    b. Over the xiphoid process
    c. Over the sternum
    d. Over the trachea

65. The iliac crests of the pelvis are palpated by gentle compression posteriorly and:
    a. Anteriorly
    b. Medially
    c. Laterally
    d. Superiorly

66. When examining the lower extremities, you should compare:
    a. One to the other
    b. Upper thigh to lower leg
    c. Them to the upper extremities
    d. Anterior-posterior diameter to the lateral diameter

67. The posterior tibial pulse is located behind the:
    a. Inner ankle bone (medial malleolus)
    b. Midthigh region
    c. Hip region
    d. Kneecap

68. The bone that can be palpated on the anterior surface of the lower leg is the:
    a. Humerus
    b. Tibia
    c. Fibula
    d. Femur

69. The pulse that can be palpated in the anterolateral aspect of the wrist just below the thumb is the:
    a. Brachial
    b. Ulnar
    c. Radial
    d. Humeral

70. Which of the following problems is most likely to result in an absent pulse in one arm?
    a. A shock state with decreased perfusion
    b. An obstruction of an artery by a bone end
    c. Hypotension caused by arterial constriction
    d. Failure of the left side of the heart

71. Having the patient flex and extend the foot, lift the leg, and wiggle the toes most directly evaluates:
    a. Sensory function
    b. Mental state
    c. Motor function
    d. Brainstem function

72. Which of the following patients might receive a rapid trauma assessment and be immediately transported without further physical examination?
    a. Patient with injuries to the upper arm
    b. Patient with multiple abrasions on the chest and abdomen
    c. Stable patient with fluid exuding from the nose
    d. Patient with a large chest wound and severe shock

73. What is the reason for reconsidering the mechanism of injury during the focused (secondary) assessment (history and physical examination)?
    a. To verify your initial assessment findings.
    b. The patient may have provided incorrect information.
    c. To help anticipate injury patterns during your examination.
    d. It should be reconsidered every 3 to 5 minutes.

74. The OPQRST mnemonic is most suited for a patient presenting with which type of "history of presenting illness"?
    a. Patient with a behavioral emergency
    b. Patient with an obstetric emergency
    c. Patient who sustained an environmental emergency
    d. Patient with a cardiac emergency

75. Which of the following questions represents the best way to ask a patient about the quality and nature of his or her chest pain or discomfort?
    a. Is the pain or discomfort squeezing in nature?
    b. Does it feel like a vise on your chest wall?
    c. How would you describe the pain or discomfort?
    d. Is the pain or discomfort strong or weak?

76. A useful method to have the patient describe the severity of chest pain or discomfort is:
    a. In terms of being minor, moderate, or severe.
    b. To compare it to other types of pain or discomfort (e.g., toothache).
    c. On a scale from 1 to 10.
    d. In relation to a pinch on the arm.

77. A focused (secondary) assessment (physical examination) for a patient complaining of difficulty breathing might include all the following *except:*
    a. Jugular venous distention
    b. Tenderness in the upper legs
    c. Breath sounds
    d. Swelling of the ankles

78. You respond to a call for a small child who cut her index finger on the sharp edge of a toy. What should the focused (secondary) assessment consist of?
    a. Examination of the finger and hand
    b. Examination of the finger, head, and neck
    c. Examination of the finger, head, neck, and trunk
    d. Comprehensive head-to-toe survey

79. You find a 5-year-old boy who has fallen from a height of 6 feet. The initial (primary) assessment and the focused (secondary) assessment revealed no positive findings. What should the detailed physical examination consist of?
   a. An examination of only the back side of the patient
   b. An examination of only the head and neck
   c. An examination of only the head, neck, and trunk
   d. A complete head-to-toe survey
80. You note blood drainage from the ear during a focused (secondary) assessment. What actions should you take?
   a. Place the patient's head lower than the torso.
   b. Place the patient in the lateral recumbent position.
   c. Pack the ear with soft gauze.
   d. Cover the ear with a loose dressing.
81. During the focused (secondary) assessment, you note liquid secretions collecting in the airway of an unconscious blunt trauma patient and hear gurgling sounds emitting from the airway. What action should you take?
   a. Transport the patient in the prone position.
   b. Suction the patient's airway.
   c. Perform a finger sweep.
   d. Turn the head to the side.
82. You note cyanosis of the lips and nail beds in a conscious and alert patient during your focused (secondary) assessment. What action(s) should you take?
   a. Reassess the airway, ventilation, and oxygenation of the patient.
   b. Immediately start positive-pressure ventilation with a bag-mask.
   c. Administer oxygen by nasal cannula and continue your examination.
   d. Elevate the patient's legs to ensure perfusion to the upper body.
83. During your focused (secondary) assessment, you note an impaled object in the patient's thigh. What action(s) should you take?
   a. Remove the object and apply a dressing to the area.
   b. Remove the object and irrigate the area to prevent infection.
   c. Leave the object in place and transport immediately.
   d. Stabilize the object in place with a bulky dressing.
84. Which of the following patients would *not* receive a focused (secondary) assessment?
   a. A conscious patient who fell from a height of 10 feet
   b. A stable automobile trauma patient
   c. A patient with multiple dog bites
   d. A patient in cardiopulmonary arrest

85. The focused (secondary) assessment is usually performed:
   a. At the scene before transport
   b. In the ambulance during transport
   c. Just before the initial (primary) assessment
   d. At the hospital before transferring the patient
86. Which is the most important reason for rechecking vitals signs during the ongoing assessment?
   a. The patient's condition may have deteriorated since your last evaluation.
   b. To confirm the accuracy of the reading previously taken by your partner.
   c. To ensure effective medical and legal documentation for the record.
   d. To reassure the patient that he or she is receiving the best possible treatment.
87. Sequential blood pressures of 120/80, 110/76, and 90/60 mm Hg were discovered during your ongoing assessment of a trauma patient. Which of the following would best explain this pattern?
   a. Normal variance in a healthy patient.
   b. Changes caused by severe anxiety.
   c. Calming of the patient related to oxygen therapy.
   d. Trending during uncontrolled internal bleeding.
88. During the transport of a patient who was complaining of difficulty breathing, you reassess vital signs and note the following: the patient's mental state changes from alert and oriented to responsive to painful stimuli; his pulse rate increases from 80 to 110 beats/min; and his respiratory rate changes from 12 breaths/min and regular to 24 breaths/min and shallow. What is the value of this information to the physician at the emergency department?
   a. It demonstrates marked improvement in the patient's condition.
   b. It indicates that the patient is stable and responding to treatment.
   c. It shows that the patient is getting worse.
   d. It indicates that the patient requires minimal additional treatment.
89. You are administering oxygen by nonrebreather mask to a patient complaining of chest pain and note the following during your ongoing assessment en route to the hospital. The patient becomes cyanotic and unresponsive, respiratory rate is 8 breaths/min and shallow, and pulse is 120 beats/min and thready. What immediate action should you take?
   a. Increase the oxygen concentration.
   b. Elevate the patient's head.
   c. Administer abdominal thrusts.
   d. Administer positive-pressure ventilation.

90. You are transporting a patient with a traction splint. What specific evaluation would be most appropriate during your ongoing assessment or reassessment?
   a. Measure the circumference of the injured extremity.
   b. Check for a distal pulse in the injured extremity.
   c. Test for tenderness by palpating the injured extremity.
   d. Lift the extremity and check for edema in the posterior region.

91. An effective method for evaluating changes in the severity of chest pain or discomfort during your ongoing assessment or reassessment is to:
   a. Have the patient rate the pain or discomfort on a scale of 1 to 10.
   b. Have the patient use an appropriate adjective to describe severity.
   c. Apply painful stimuli, and have the patient compare the two stimuli.
   d. Have the patient compare the pain or discomfort to another unrelated event.

92. The ongoing assessment or reassessment is started by:
   a. A review of the initial assessment.
   b. Examination of the head.
   c. Checking the blood pressure.
   d. Checking skin temperature.

93. As a general rule, how often should *unstable* patients be reassessed during your ongoing assessment?
   a. Every 1 minute
   b. Every 5 minutes
   c. Every 10 minutes
   d. Every 15 minutes

94. As a general rule, how often should *stable* patients be reassessed during your ongoing assessment?
   a. Every 1 minute
   b. Every 5 minutes
   c. Every 10 minutes
   d. Every 15 minutes

MATCHING

Match the respiratory sound in column A with the likely underlying problem in column B.

Column A	Column B
_____ 95. Gurgling	a. Obstruction by the tongue
_____ 96. Snoring	b. Fluid in the airway
_____ 97. Wheezing	c. Narrowed lower airway
_____ 98. Stridor	d. Narrowed upper airway

FILL IN THE BLANK

99. The measure of the force that blood exerts on the walls of the arteries is called _____ _____.

100. The membrane of the interior surface of the eyelids, used to assess skin color, is the _____.

101. A blood pressure should be taken in children above _____ years of age.

102. _____ is the mnemonic used to stay organized during your history taking.

103. An exaggerated opening of the nostrils on inspiration, which is a sign of respiratory distress seen in infants and children, is called _____ _____.

104. _____ are inward depressions of muscular areas between the ribs, above the clavicles, and below the sternum seen in a patient in respiratory distress.

105. You respond to a motor vehicle incident on a country road outside town. Your initial scene size-up reveals that two cars have been involved in a head-on collision at a high rate of speed. There are five patients in one car and three patients in the other car. One vehicle is leaking gasoline, and a puddle is spreading down the roadway. Based on the number of patients involved in this incident, you would initiate your department's _____ _____ _____ plan.

106. Posterior _____ of the hip causes the leg to rotate internally, adduct, and flex at the knee.

107. A physical finding in the neck that may indicate a backup of blood in the venous system returning to the heart is called _____ _____ _____.

108. The forces that might have injured the trauma patient are called the _____ _____ _____.

109. The mnemonic used during the rapid trauma assessment to remember possible physical findings during the head-to-toe survey is _____.

110. Injured sections of the thorax moving in opposite directions from the uninjured sections is called _____ _____.

111. Abnormal change in the position of the windpipe, suggesting injury to the airway or chest, is called _____ _____.

Questions 112-117. OPQRST is a mnemonic designed to help you remember questions that clarify the chief complaint. Fill in the appropriate word next to each letter of the mnemonic.

112. O_____

113. P _____

114. Q_____

115. R_____

116. S_____

117. T_____

118. Asking questions regarding vomiting, antacid use, and rectal bleeding would be most appropriate for a patient presenting with the chief complaint of

    _____ _____.

119. During the focused (secondary) assessment, a penlight is used to examine the eyes to check if

    the pupils _____ when exposed to light.

120. A contusion or black-and-blue discoloration

    behind the ear may be a sign of a _____

    _____.

121. To control bleeding from the nose, pinch the nose

    with the patient leaning _____ if conditions permit.

122. The ongoing assessment or reassessment of the patient's responsiveness should be completed

    quickly with the mnemonic _____.

123. The best visual indicator of an open airway and sufficient breathing is to observe for adequate

    _____ _____.

124. Empathy and providing emotional support are especially significant in children and

    _____ _____.

SHORT ANSWER

Questions 125-130. List the six questions that you should ask the patient with an obstetric emergency.

125. _____

    _____

126. _____

    _____

127. _____

    _____

128. _____

    _____

129. _____

    _____

130. _____

    _____

Questions 131-135. List the five key questions to ask the patient or yourself with a behavioral emergency.

131. _____

    _____

132. _____

    _____

133. _____

    _____

134. _____

    _____

135. _____

    _____

Questions 136-141. List the six key questions to ask the patient with a poisoning/overdose.

136. _____

    _____

137. _____

    _____

138. _____

    _____

139. _____

    _____

140. _____

    _____

141. _____

    _____

Questions 142-149. List the eight key questions to ask the patient or bystander, or things to look for, in a patient with an altered level of consciousness.

142. _____

    _____

143. _____

    _____

144. _____

    _____

145. _____

    _____

146. _____

    _____

147. _____

148. _____

149. _____

Questions 150-155. List the six key questions to ask the patient with an allergic reaction.

150. _____

151. _____

152. _____

153. _____

154. _____

155. _____

Questions 156-160. List the five key questions to ask the patient, or things to look for, in a patient with an environmental emergency.

156. _____

157. _____

158. _____

159. _____

160. _____

Qustions 161-164. List the four key components of the ongoing assessment or reassessment.

161. _____

162. _____

163. _____

164. _____

Questions 165-167. List three abnormal skin colors and a common reason for each physical finding.

165. _____

166. _____

167. _____

TRUE/FALSE

168. _____ Requesting additional resources to the scene of the incident is part of the scene size-up.

169. _____ The detailed physical assessment should be completed during the scene size-up.

170. _____ The most common hazard encountered by the EMT is the traffic surrounding auto incidents.

171. _____ The use of flares as a traffic delineation device is most beneficial in the daytime.

172. _____ When responding to a violent call, such as a shooting, you should approach the scene as soon as possible and initiate care while awaiting police arrival.

173. _____ Reconstructing the forces of injury helps the EMT to anticipate potential injuries.

174. _____ Patient triage and initial (primary) assessment of the patient should be instituted before ensuring scene safety.

175. _____ Self-contained breathing apparatus should be worn when treating a patient with suspected tuberculosis.

176. _____ A multiple-casualty incident plan should be initiated only after an emergency medical services supervisor has responded to the scene and assessed the situation.

177. _____ A rapid trauma assessment must be performed on every trauma patient, no matter how minor or severe the injury appears.

178. _____ A patient who lacerated her thumb while cutting a bagel requires a focused (secondary) assessment (physical exam) of the hand; a rapid trauma assessment is not required.

179. _____ Dentures that are stable should be left in place.

180. _____ The detailed physical examination is performed more rapidly than the initial (primary) assessment and focused examination.

181. _____ The scalp is very vascular, and small injuries may present with extensive bleeding.

Questions 182 to 186 refer to the following scenario.
You respond to the scene of a patient who fell off a roof. On arrival you find a 27-year-old man lying supine in the driveway. The fire department has secured the area, and the scene is safe. A neighbor advises you that the patient was on the roof, approximately 15 feet high, when he stumbled backward and fell to the driveway, striking the back of his head. You and your partner have taken proper body substance isolation precautions.

182. While you check the patient for responsiveness, you should direct your partner to:
    a. Open the airway with a head-tilt/chin-lift maneuver.
    b. Manually stabilize the cervical spine.
    c. Log-roll the patient onto his left side to maintain an open airway.
    d. Quickly lift the patient onto your stretcher in preparation for rapid transport.

183. You initially ask the patient if he is all right. There is no response, and you ask again, in a loud voice, "Are you OK?" The patient responds by groaning. Based on this response, you would place him in which AVPU category?
    a. A
    b. V
    c. P
    d. U

184. Evaluation of your patient reveals that he is breathing at approximately 14 breaths/min without use of accessory muscles, and there is adequate chest expansion with each breath. Supplemental oxygen:
    a. Is not required at this time.
    b. Should be administered by a bag-mask device.
    c. Should be administered by a nasal cannula at 4 to 6 L/min.
    d. Should be administered by a nonrebreather mask at 15 L/min.

185. After checking for responsiveness, airway, and breathing, you would check for circulation by feeling for a pulse at the:
    a. Carotid artery
    b. Femoral artery
    c. Radial artery
    d. Temporal artery

186. You assess whether this patient requires early transportation and determine that:
    a. Early transportation is not indicated because the patient is not unconscious.
    b. Early transportation is not indicated because the patient has a patent airway.
    c. Early transportation is indicated because the patient fell approximately 15 feet.
    d. Early transportation is indicated because the patient has an altered mental status.

Questions 187 to 189 refer to the following scenario.
You are called to the scene of a bicycle rider who was struck by a car. The police have secured the area, and the scene is safe. You and your partner have taken appropriate body substance isolation precautions. You encounter a 16-year-old girl who is sitting on the curb. She is alert, complaining of pain in her back; her airway, breathing, and circulation are all normal.

187. This patient requires a:
    a. Rapid trauma assessment, performed on the scene, because of the mechanism of injury.
    b. Rapid trauma assessment, performed in the ambulance, because of the mechanism of injury.
    c. Focused physical examination of the patient's back because of an isolated chief complaint.
    d. Detailed physical examination performed immediately.

188. Spinal immobilization of this patient is:
    a. Not needed because the patient reported that she walked after the incident.
    b. Only indicated if the assessment reveals neurologic damage.
    c. Immediately indicated and should be performed as soon as possible.
    d. Indicated but should not be done until all the assessment steps are completed.

189. On evaluation, you determine that the patient complains of pain on palpation of her lower back. Using the DCAP/BTLS mnemonic, you would document that the patient has _____ to her lower back.
    a. a contusion
    b. an abrasion
    c. tenderness
    d. swelling

Questions 190 to 193 refer to the following scenario.
You are transporting a 57-year-old man to the hospital. The patient's chief complaint is chest pressure that he describes as "constant" and rates a 5 on a 10-point pain scale. The patient's skin color looks yellow, and he tells you he has liver disease. You have administered oxygen, and your transport time is 12 minutes. After a few minutes of receiving oxygen, the patient informs you that his chest pressure is now a 3 on a 10-point scale.

190. The reason to reevaluate your patient's pain and rate it on a pain scale is:
    a. To determine your patient's tolerance for pain.
    b. To determine when the oxygen can be removed.
    c. To determine if your treatment is having any effect.
    d. To determine the appropriate position to transport the patient.

191. The yellow skin color that you observe in your patient is called:
    a. Cyanosis
    b. Pallor
    c. Mottled
    d. Jaundice

192. Your ongoing assessment of this patient while en route to the hospital includes all of the following *except:*
    a. Repeat of the vital signs.
    b. Repeat of the initial (primary) assessment.
    c. Reevaluation of the patient's chest discomfort.
    d. SAMPLE history (signs and symptoms, allergies, medications, past medical problems, last oral intake, events surrounding this illness).

193. Your patient is concerned about his condition, and he asks you if he is having a heart attack. You should inform him that:
    a. He is not having a heart attack, and he should remain calm.
    b. His symptoms indicate that he is having a heart attack, but you are there to help him.
    c. You are not able to diagnose his problem, but you are providing the best possible care for him based on his symptoms.
    d. You are not allowed to comment on his condition until he is evaluated by a physician at the hospital.

CROSSWORD PUZZLE

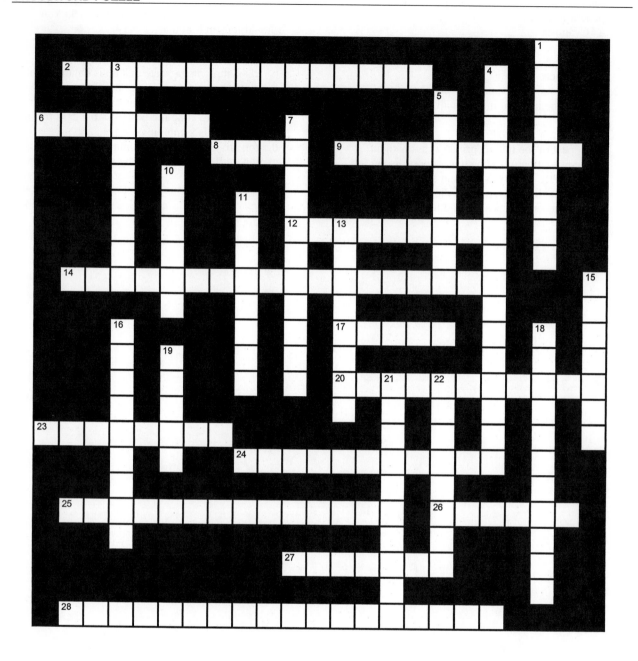

Across

2. Assessment performed on a patient who is unresponsive or has an altered mental status
6. Subjective description of the complaint in the patient's own words
8. How long the problem has existed
9. The T in DCAP/BTLS
12. Pain that spreads to another body part or area
14. Respirations, pulse, blood pressure, and mental state
17. The B in DCAP/BTLS
20. The L in DCAP/BTLS
23. The L in SAMPLE
24. The M in SAMPLE
25. Relevant information associated with the chief complaint
26. The E in SAMPLE
27. Frequently the most significant part of patient assessment
28. Information regarding previous illnesses and hospitalizations and current medications

Down

1. The A in DCAP/BTLS
3. The A in SAMPLE
4. The S in SAMPLE
5. The S in DCAP/BTLS
7. The D in DCAP/BTLS
10. Mnemonic to remember the key questions in a patient history
11. Degree of pain
13. Mnemonic used to remember possible physical findings identified during the head-to-toe survey
15. Examination directed toward the chief complaint
16. The P in DCAP/BTLS
18. Behaviors that make the symptoms better or worse
19. When the complaint first occurred
21. The C in DCAP/BTLS
22. Position used for an unresponsive medical patient to protect the airway during transport

8 | Communications

MULTIPLE CHOICE

1. When initiating a radio call, the EMT should:
   a. Interrupt radio transmission that is in progress.
   b. Ask permission to interrupt radio transmission that is in progress.
   c. Use the squelch feature on the radio to interrupt any radio transmission in the event of an emergency.
   d. Never interrupt a radio transmission.

2. The most effective way to begin your radio transmission is to:
   a. Identify yourself and your unit.
   b. Present the patient's chief complaint.
   c. Present the patient's vital signs.
   d. Present the patient's past medical history.

3. At the end of each verbal radio exchange, the speaker should end the message with the word(s):
   a. "Next."
   b. "Over."
   c. "Message complete."
   d. "Roger."

4. When initiating a radio call, the EMT should:
   a. Wait for the receiving unit to say "go ahead" before sending the message.
   b. Use "yes" and "no" to indicate acceptance or refusal of the response.
   c. Speak in a voice that is louder than normal.
   d. Consider using codes to reduce on-air time and summarize communications.

5. Which of the following is the typical medical format used for presenting a patient?
   a. Estimated time of arrival, patient's name, and vital signs
   b. Patient's age, gender, and history of present illness (chief complaint)
   c. EMS unit identifier, patient's vital signs, and estimated time of arrival
   d. Patient's physician's name, history of present illness (chief complaint), and estimated time of arrival

6. The typical medical format for presenting a patient should conclude with:
   a. Patient's name, age, and gender
   b. Prehospital treatments rendered and patient's response
   c. EMS identifier, patient's history of present illness (chief complaint), and past medical history
   d. EMS identifier, estimated time of arrival, and EMT's diagnosis of patient's condition

7. Which of the following statements is true?
   a. When giving your report, accuracy is essential.
   b. When giving your report, accuracy is not essential because the hospital will reassess the patient once you arrive.
   c. The EMT is responsible for making a prehospital diagnosis.
   d. The EMT should give a lengthy, presumptive report over the radio.

8. Which of the following statements is true?
   a. The dispatcher will always notify the receiving hospital.
   b. The dispatcher will never notify the receiving hospital.
   c. The information you provide is essential in preparing the hospital for your arrival.
   d. The information you provide is of no value in preparing the hospital for your arrival.

9. A good rule to follow when speaking into a radio microphone is to:
   a. Talk louder than normal while holding the microphone right next to your mouth.
   b. Speak in a normal voice with the microphone a few inches away from your mouth.
   c. Speak more slowly than normal and in a low voice.
   d. Speak in a normal voice with the microphone touching your mouth.

10. As a general rule, how many inches should the microphone be held away from your mouth while speaking?
    a. 2 to 3
    b. 5 to 6
    c. 8 to 10
    d. 10 to 12

11. As a rule, radio communication allows for:
    a. Both parties to speak at the same time.
    b. One person to speak at a time.
    c. Interruption for a more serious patient.
    d. A dispatcher to connect both parties.

12. The governmental agency responsible for regulating all aspects of radio communication in the United States is called the:
    a. Radio Communications Center (RCC)
    b. Dispatch Communications Center (DCC)
    c. Federal Communications Commission (FCC)
    d. Center for Federal Communications (CFC)

13. Focusing your attention on the patient, telling the truth, and using language the patient will understand are all components of:
    a. The standard medical presentation format
    b. The governmental agency that regulates radio communications in the United States
    c. The primary assessment
    d. Interpersonal communication skills
14. Speaking clearly, slowly, and distinctly and using the patient's proper name are examples of:
    a. Nonverbal communication skills
    b. Verbal communication skills
    c. Body communication skills
    d. Radio communication skills
15. Which of the following may be appropriate when communicating with a patient who speaks another language?
    a. Shout in a very loud voice.
    b. Do not attempt any further communication until you arrive at the hospital.
    c. Use a translator if one is available and time permits.
    d. Do not initiate transport until a translator arrives at the scene.
16. It is appropriate to use medical terms when communicating with:
    a. The patient
    b. The patient's family
    c. Other EMTs
    d. Bystanders

SHORT ANSWER

Questions 17-19. List three special problems or techniques that the EMT may encounter or perform when dealing with elderly patients.

17. _____

    _____

18. _____

    _____

19. _____

    _____

Questions 20-23. List four special problems or techniques that the EMT may encounter or perform when dealing with the sick or injured child.

20. _____

    _____

21. _____

    _____

22. _____

    _____

23. _____

    _____

Questions 24-27. List four special problems or techniques that the EMT may encounter or perform when dealing with a deaf patient.

24. _____

    _____

25. _____

    _____

26. _____

    _____

27. _____

    _____

Questions 28-30. List three special problems or techniques that the EMT may encounter or perform when dealing with a blind patient.

28. _____

    _____

29. _____

    _____

30. _____

    _____

Questions 31-35. List five special problems or techniques that the EMT may encounter or perform when dealing with a confused patient.

31. _____

    _____

32. _____

    _____

33. _____

    _____

34. _____

    _____

35. _____

    _____

Questions 36-39. List four special problems or techniques that the EMT may encounter or perform when dealing with patients who are mentally challenged.

36. _____

    _____

37. _____

    _____

38. _____

   _____

39. _____

   _____

CASE SCENARIO

Questions 40 to 42 refer to the following scenario.
You are called to respond to the local community college, where you encounter a 19-year-old woman who was stung by a bee. The patient tells you that her sister is allergic to bees, and the patient is afraid that she also might be allergic. She has some slight swelling on her arm at the site of the sting but no other complaints.

40. You call medical control and speak with a physician to determine if you should administer an EpiPen to this patient. This type of communication is called:
   a. Online medical control
   b. Offline medical control
   c. Standing orders
   d. Protocols

41. In the past, your radio communication system from your ambulance to the base physician has not been reliable because of poor signal strength. The recent addition of a _____ to your radio system boosts the signal strength and allows for more reliable communications.

42. As you are concluding your call with the base physician, a local taxicab company begins to break into your radio communication. You are concerned that this type of radio interference could jeopardize emergency communications, and you report this incident to your supervisor. Your supervisor reports this incident to the governmental agency responsible for regulating radio communications in the United States. This agency is the:
   a. Center for Radio Control (CRC)
   b. Emergency Medical Services Dispatching Coordinator (EMSDC)
   c. Frequency Allocation Agency (FAA)
   d. Federal Communications Commission (FCC)

9 Documentation

1. The narrative section of the written prehospital care report is used to:
   a. Relay the facts regarding how you found the patient.
   b. Definitively conclude what happened to the patient.
   c. Document the radio codes used on the call.
   d. Record the patient's vital signs.

2. Effective record keeping includes the systematic collection of data from the dispatch phase through the transfer of care to the emergency department staff. Which of the following information is *least* desirable?
   a. Location of the call
   b. Name of the person calling for assistance
   c. Patient assessment
   d. Changes in patient condition

3. In what section of the prehospital care report are the patient's chief complaint, level of consciousness, and blood pressure recorded?
   a. Assessment data
   b. Treatment data
   c. Patient disposition
   d. Run data

4. In what section of the prehospital care report is the application of a splint documented?
   a. Patient disposition
   b. Run data
   c. Patient data
   d. Treatment data

5. In what section of the prehospital care report is the receiving hospital and emergency department staff member accepting the patient documented?
   a. Patient disposition
   b. Run data
   c. Patient data
   d. Treatment data

6. The information ascertained during the treatment of the patient, such as vital signs, is part of the:
   a. Dispatch data
   b. Patient data
   c. Assessment data
   d. Treatment data

7. Most emergency medical services systems use military times to document the respective phases of a call. In military time, 3 PM is expressed as:
   a. 1300 hours
   b. 1400 hours
   c. 1500 hours
   d. 1600 hours

8. Noon is expressed in military time as:
   a. 0000 hours
   b. 1200 hours
   c. 2400 hours
   d. 0100 hours

9. Which of the following represents the *best* or objective documentation of a suspected case of alcohol intoxication on an ambulance call report?
   a. The patient appeared intoxicated with an alcohol-like compound.
   b. There was an alcohol-like smell on the patient's breath.
   c. The patient was speaking as if he was intoxicated.
   d. The patient was extremely intoxicated.

10. Which of these statements is *least* effective when documenting biological death in the patient data section of the written prehospital care report?
    a. The patient was dead for 30 minutes before our arrival.
    b. The patient has extreme dependent lividity on the back and posterior legs.
    c. The patient has evidence of rigor mortis in all extremities.
    d. The patient has sustained severe destruction of the skull and brain from the fall.

11. The effectiveness of a written prehospital care report depends on which of the following four major factors?
    a. Accuracy, clarity, chronology, completeness
    b. Legibility, clarity, judgment, accuracy
    c. Clarity, accuracy, completeness, judgment
    d. Legibility, honesty, accuracy, completeness

12. The refusal signature is of no value unless the EMT:
    a. Informs the patient of the potential consequences of refusal.
    b. Has at least two copies of the refusal.
    c. Has a police officer witness the refusal.
    d. Has rendered at least some first-aid care.

13. Which of the following people is *least* effective as a witness to refusal of care?
    a. Patient's family member
    b. Bystander
    c. EMT partner
    d. Police officer

14. The EMT can share the information about a patient's condition with:
    a. The general public
    b. Only a friend
    c. Reporters as requested
    d. Emergency department staff as documented

59

15. Which of the following patients has the right to refuse medical aid?
    a. Unconscious patient with history of diabetes
    b. Competent adult patient with wrist injury
    c. Six-year-old girl struck by car
    d. Diabetic patient with altered level of consciousness
16. If you are treating a patient who is a minor without a parent or guardian present or is unconscious, it is best to:
    a. Render care to your level of training and transport the patient.
    b. Withhold transport until a relative can be located.
    c. Have a bystander accompany the patient to the hospital.
    d. Transport the patient with a police officer.
17. Reviewing written prehospital care reports to evaluate effectiveness of prehospital care is called:
    a. Legal protection
    b. Peer review
    c. Continuing education
    d. Continuous quality improvement
18. When an error of omission occurs, the EMT should:
    a. Falsify the information on the written prehospital care report.
    b. Document what would have been done according to local protocol.
    c. Rewrite the written prehospital care report to reflect what should have happened.
    d. Document what actually did or did not happen and what steps, if any, were taken to correct the situation.
19. To correct an error that occurs while writing the prehospital care report, you should:
    a. Obliterate the error and start over.
    b. Draw a single horizontal line through the error, initial, and rewrite with the correct information.
    c. Draw two diagonal lines forming an X through the error, initial, and rewrite with the correct information.
    d. Destroy all copies and start over.

FILL IN THE BLANK

Questions 20-41. Insert the abbreviation or symbol for the following terms.

20. Male _____
21. Female _____
22. Before _____
23. Blood pressure _____
24. With _____
25. Complaining of _____
26. Cardiopulmonary resuscitation _____
27. Date of birth _____
28. History _____
29. Left lower quadrant _____
30. Left upper quadrant _____
31. Nitroglycerin _____
32. Oxygen _____
33. By mouth _____
34. Patient _____
35. Physical examination _____
36. Right lower quadrant _____
37. Right upper quadrant _____
38. Sublingual _____
39. Shortness of breath _____
40. Treatment _____
41. Years old _____

CASE SCENARIO

Questions 42 and 43 refer to the following scenario.
You are dispatched to a call at 2355 hours to care for a patient with injuries from a fall. On arrival you find a 15-year-old boy who injured his left thumb when he tripped and fell. The patient is staying with a 16-year-old friend; there are no adults present. The patient tells you that the injury is "nothing much," and that he will wait until his parents arrive in about 2 hours.

42. You arrive at the scene of this call at 10 minutes after midnight. The proper way to document this time is:
    a. 12:10 AM
    b. 0010 hours
    c. 2410 hours
    d. 0110 hours
43. This patient wants to refuse aid. You know that:
    a. The patient can refuse aid because he is an emancipated minor.
    b. The patient must be treated under the concept of implied consent because of the injury and transported to the hospital.
    c. The patient is a minor and cannot refuse medical aid.
    d. The friend can sign the refusal for the patient.

CROSSWORD PUZZLE

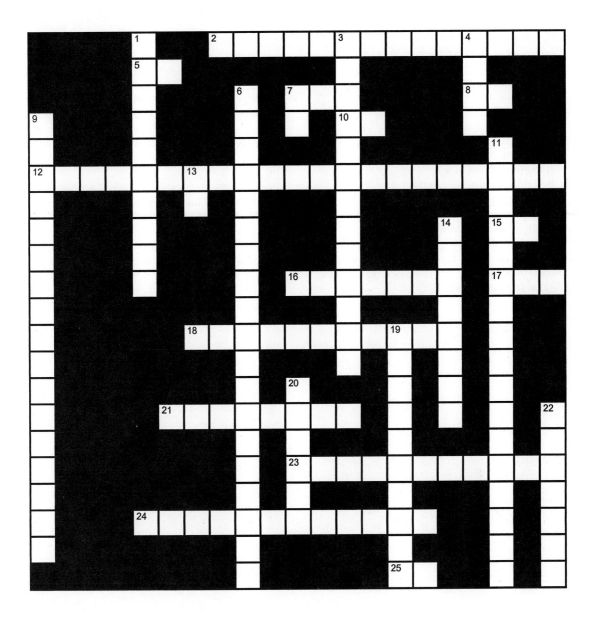

Across

2. The expression of the patient's main problem in his or her own words
5. History (abbreviation)
7. "Bag-valve-mask" (abbreviation; corect term now *bag-mask*)
8. By mouth (abbreviation)
10. Physical examination (abbreviation)
12. A medical record and legal document that is a complete record of a call
15. Treatment (abbreviation)
16. Information regarding the dispatch of a call
17. Nitroglycerin (abbreviation)
18. Muscle rigidity following death
21. _____ and honesty are vital in avoiding jeopardizing care of patients.
23. Demographic information about the victim
24. No information should be given to anyone other than essential personnel regarding the patient's condition because it is _____.
25. Sublingual (abbreviation)

Down

1. Time relationships
3. c/o
4. Mnemonic used to remember the assessment of a patient's mental status
6. Call review sessions are a primary means of _____ _____ for EMTs.
7. Blood pressure (abbreviation)
9. Mottling of the dependent areas of the body
11. _____ _____ improvement reports are reviewed to evaluate the effectiveness of prehospital care.
13. Patient (abbreviation)
14. y/o
19. During a disaster, _____ _____ are used for notation of a patient's status.
20. Mnemonic to remember the key questions in a patient's history
22. PCRs should be written with _____ so that they are easily understood by the reader.

10 General Pharmacology

MULTIPLE CHOICE

1. Which of the following prescribed medications may an EMT assist with administering when a patient has the medication available?
   a. Epinephrine
   b. Atropine
   c. Digoxin
   d. Lidocaine
2. A simple form of the chemical name of a medication is called the:
   a. Trade name
   b. Biochemical name
   c. Basic name
   d. Generic name
3. Situations in which a drug should *not* be used because it may cause harm to the patient or have no effect is called a(n):
   a. Side effect
   b. Complication
   c. Contraindication
   d. Adverse reaction
4. What is a common route of administration for nitroglycerin?
   a. Intramuscular
   b. Sublingual
   c. Intravenous
   d. Inhaler
5. Which of the following doses is equivalent to 1 g?
   a. 10 mg
   b. 100 mg
   c. 1000 mg
   d. 1000 mmcg
6. What is a key consideration when administering activated charcoal?
   a. Drinking it very slowly to ensure absorption.
   b. Mixing it with milk to create the appropriate mixture.
   c. Drinking 2 teaspoons at a time.
   d. Shaking it before administration.
7. The effects of a drug on organs other than the desired action are called:
   a. Adverse reactions
   b. Side effects
   c. Contraindications
   d. Complications
8. Which of the following patients is most likely to be a candidate for glucose administration?
   a. Patient who is dehydrated
   b. Patient who is vomiting
   c. Patient with suspected hypoglycemia
   d. Patient with chest pain

MATCHING

Questions 9-13. Match the name of a drug in column B to the correct form of the drug in column A.

Column A	Column B
9. _____ Tablet	a. Activated charcoal
10. _____ Suspension	b. Epinephrine
11. _____ Gel	c. Oxygen
12. _____ Liquid for injection	d. Nitroglycerin
13. _____ Gas	e. Oral glucose

Questions 14-20. Match the drug names in column A with their type in column B.

Column A	Column B
14. _____ Glucose	a. Generic
15. _____ EpiPen	b. Trade
16. _____ Actidose	
17. _____ Alupent	
18. _____ Nitrostat	
19. _____ Epinephrine	
20. _____ Albuterol	

FILL IN THE BLANK

Questions 21-25. Write a word in the blank to complete the sentence.

21. The science that deals with the origin, nature, chemistry, effects, and uses of drugs is called

    _____.

22. A _____ is any chemical compound that may be administered to someone as an aid in the treatment or improvement of an abnormal condition.

23. A child weighs 22 lb. How many kilograms does this child weigh? _____

24. The medication carried on the ambulance, often packaged as a suspension, that may be used to treat certain suspected toxic ingestions at the direction of medical control, is called _____ _____.

25. One liter (1 L) of fluid contains _____ mL.

SHORT ANSWER

Questions 26-30. List the five "rights" of medication administration.

26. _____

    _____

27. _____

_____

28. _____

_____

29. _____

_____

30. _____

_____

CASE SCENARIOS

Questions 31 to 33 refer to the following scenario.
You are called to the scene of an attempted suicide. The scene is secured, and the police are present. Your patient is a 16-year-old girl who tells you that she wanted to kill herself and that she took 20 tablets of acetaminophen, each containing 500 mg. The patient weighs 110 pounds. At present the patient is stable with a pulse rate of 80 beats/min, blood pressure of 116/72 mm Hg, and respiratory rate of 16 breaths/min.

31. As per your protocol, you call the regional poison control center to determine if any interventions should be initiated on the scene. The nurse specialist on the phone asks you to calculate the patient's weight in kilograms so that they can determine if the quantity of medication taken is at the toxic level. This patient weighs:
    a. 40 kg
    b. 50 kg
    c. 60 kg
    d. 70 kg
32. You would anticipate that the poison control center would advise you to:
    a. Administer an EpiPen.
    b. Administer an EpiPen Jr.
    c. Provide emotional and medical support for the patient and transport her to the hospital.
    d. Induce vomiting by placing your gloved finger in the back of the patient's mouth.
33. Albuterol is a:
    a. Trade name
    b. Biochemical name
    c. Basic name
    d. Generic name

Questions 34 to 36 refer to the following scenario.
You respond to a call in an apartment complex and find a 53-year-old man complaining of left-sided chest pressure that radiates down his left arm. The patient appears pale and sweaty. The patient has a cardiac history and has a bottle of nitroglycerin with him. He has not taken the nitroglycerin, and you note that the medication is prescribed to him and is not out of date. The patient has a blood pressure of 156/88 mm Hg, heart rate of 88 beats/min and regular, and respiratory rate of 14 breaths/min. The patient tells you that he is not allergic to anything, that his only past medical history is a heart attack 2 years ago, and that he took Viagra about 1 hour ago.

34. In this scenario you would *not* assist this patient in taking a nitroglycerin tablet because you know that Viagra may interact with the nitroglycerin and produce unwanted and possibly harmful effects. This is called a(n):
    a. Contraindication
    b. Complication
    c. Side effect
    d. Adverse reaction
35. After the call is over, you critique the call with your partner and review the reasons for *not* assisting the patient in taking nitroglycerin. Your partner, who is studying to be an EMT, tells you that on a previous call a patient took a nitroglycerin tablet but then complained of a headache. You tell your partner that the patient's headache was:
    a. A contraindication in taking the drug
    b. A complication in taking the drug
    c. A side effect of taking the drug
    d. An adverse reaction that is life threatening
36. You remember that if you were to assist a patient in taking a nitroglycerin tablet, this medication would be administered:
    a. By a nebulizer connected to an oxygen source
    b. Rectally
    c. With an autoinjector
    d. Sublingually

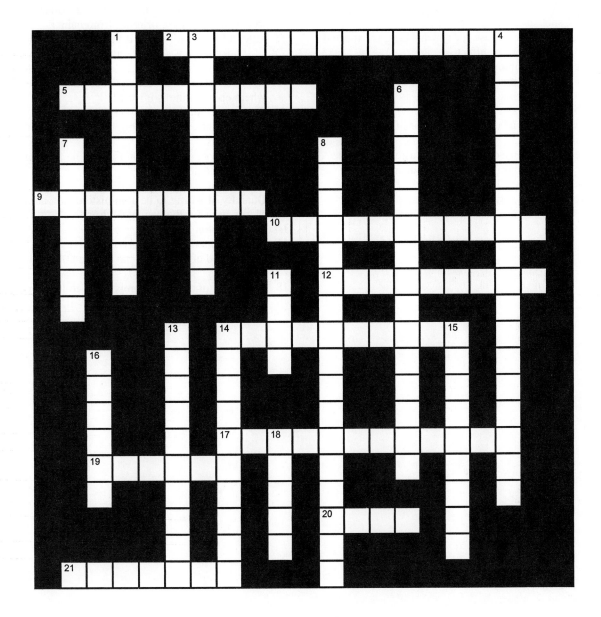

Chapter **10** **General Pharmacology**

Across

2. Common means of administering drugs through the skin, such as a nitroglycerin patch
5. A condition or disease for which a drug is expected to have a beneficial effect
9. Premeasured amounts of drug to be administered
10. The generic name for an EpiPen
12. The generic name for Ventolin
14. Solid particles mixed in a liquid
17. A way of administering medications through the bone
19. Medication carried by the EMT-Basic that is a gas
20. Method of administration of a medication by swallowing
21. Medication in spray form

Down

1. Chemical compound administered to someone for treatment of disease or relief from pain
3. After administration of a drug, a patient must be _____ for the possible effects and side effects of the drug.
4. Layer of fat and connective tissue beneath the skin where epinephrine is injected
6. The amount of drug necessary to provide the desired effect, yet low enough to minimize side effects
7. This name of a medication is a simple form of its chemical name.
8. The generic name for SuperChar
11. Quantity of a drug to be administered at one time
13. Metric term for the weight of drugs
14. Under the tongue
15. The trade name for nitroglycerin
16. The desired effect a drug has on the body or target organ
18. This name of a medication is given to it by the pharmaceutical company that makes it.

11 Respiratory Emergencies

MULTIPLE CHOICE

1. The structure that covers the trachea during swallowing to prevent aspiration is called the:
   a. Pharynx
   b. Epiglottis
   c. Thyroid cartilage
   d. Cricoid cartilage

2. The respiratory structure that is palpable just above the sternum is the:
   a. Bronchus
   b. Trachea
   c. Carina
   d. Bronchiole

3. The muscle that separates the chest and abdomen is called the:
   a. Diaphragm
   b. Intercostals
   c. Abdominis recti
   d. None of the above

4. The normal resting tidal volume for an adult is approximately:
   a. 500 mL
   b. 800 mL
   c. 1000 mL
   d. 2000 mL

5. The process by which gases move from an area of higher concentration to an area of lower concentration is called:
   a. Ventilation
   b. Respiration
   c. Diffusion
   d. Transportation

6. The portion of the lung where diffusion takes place is called the:
   a. Bronchi
   b. Pleura
   c. Bronchiole
   d. Alveoli

7. The amount of air inhaled and exhaled during a given breath is called the:
   a. Residual volume
   b. Expiratory reserve
   c. Total volume
   d. Tidal volume

8. Normal atmospheric air contains approximately what percentage of oxygen?
   a. 15%
   b. 21%
   c. 28%
   d. 50%

9. A term commonly used to describe a feeling of difficulty breathing is:
   a. Hemoptysis
   b. Tachypnea
   c. Dyspnea
   d. Ischemia

10. A bluish discoloration of the skin caused by oxygen-poor hemoglobin is called:
    a. Mottling
    b. Ecchymosis
    c. Cyanosis
    d. Anoxic erythema

11. The accessory muscles of inspiration are noted primarily by observing the:
    a. Chest wall
    b. Neck
    c. Abdominal wall
    d. Back

12. A high-pitched sound that is emitted from the lower airway that usually occurs on expiration and may be caused by asthma or chronic obstructive pulmonary disease is called:
    a. Wheezes
    b. Stridor
    c. Rhonchi
    d. Crackles

13. During positive-pressure ventilation, effective tidal volume is evaluated primarily on the basis of:
    a. Chest rise
    b. Skin color
    c. Pupil response
    d. None of the above

14. In children the most common complication of excessive or forceful ventilation is:
    a. Cyanosis
    b. Gastric distention
    c. Oxygen toxicity
    d. Air embolism

15. A patient who is exhibiting wheezing, stridor, accessory muscle use, and a weak, ineffective cough probably has a:
    a. Complete airway obstruction
    b. Partial airway obstruction with good air exchange
    c. Partial airway obstruction with poor air exchange
    d. None of the above

16. The most definitive sign of a complete airway obstruction in a conscious patient is:
    a. Cyanosis of the skin
    b. Wheezing on inspiration
    c. Snoring on expiration
    d. Inability to speak

67

17. In a pregnant woman, the correct location for a chest thrust to relieve a foreign body obstruction is:
    a. The upper portion of the sternum
    b. The sternum on the nipple line
    c. The lower half of the sternum
    d. Directly over the xiphoid process
18. If your initial attempt at ventilation is unsuccessful in an unconscious patient, your next action is to:
    a. Deliver four back blows.
    b. Deliver four abdominal thrusts.
    c. Reopen the airway and attempt ventilation.
    d. Perform a finger sweep.
19. In a child or infant with a complete airway obstruction, you should perform a finger sweep only if:
    a. The patient is conscious.
    b. The epiglottis is visible.
    c. Three attempts at ventilation are unsuccessful.
    d. You can visualize the object.
20. In which of the following patients can back blows be used in the treatment of a complete airway obstruction?
    a. Less than 1 year old
    b. 1 to 8 years old
    c. 8 to 10 years old
    d. More than 10 years old
21. A patient who is breathing rapidly and shallowly at a rate of 36 breaths/min and who is unresponsive should receive:
    a. Oxygen by nonrebreather mask
    b. Positive-pressure ventilation
    c. Oxygen by nasal cannula
    d. Oxygen by Venturi mask
22. A possible complication of high-concentration oxygen administration for a patient with chronic obstructive pulmonary disease is:
    a. Pneumothorax
    b. Pulmonary embolism
    c. Pneumonia
    d. Respiratory arrest
23. An inflammation of the alveolar spaces caused by various types of infectious organisms or by aspiration of fluid into the tracheobronchial tree is called:
    a. Pneumonia
    b. Pleurisy
    c. Pneumothorax
    d. Pulmonary embolism
24. A condition that results from air entering the pleural space and causing total or partial collapse of the lungs is called:
    a. Hemothorax
    b. Pneumothorax
    c. Pleurisy
    d. Pulmonary embolism

25. The most common breath sounds associated with a pneumothorax are:
    a. Diminished or absent sounds
    b. Wheezes
    c. Rhonchi
    d. Friction rubs
26. Immediately after inhaling the medication, the patient should:
    a. Hyperventilate several times
    b. Cough vigorously to clear airways
    c. Hold his or her breath for as long as comfortable
    d. Lay supine to facilitate absorption

MATCHING

Questions 27-32. Match the inhaler medications in column A with their drug type in column B.

Column A	Column B
27. _____ Albuterol	a. Generic
28. _____ Atrovent	b. Trade
29. _____ Ventolin	
30. _____ Alupent	
31. _____ Proventil	
32. _____ Metaproterenol	

FILL IN THE BLANK

Questions 33-41. Write a word in the blank to complete the sentence.

33. A child with epiglottitis may be found sitting upright and leaning forward with his or her weight distributed on the hands, which is known as the

    _____ position.
34. The number of breaths per minute multiplied by the quantity of air exchanged with each breath is

    called _____ _____.
35. The "colorful" term used to describe patients with

    emphysema is _____ _____.
36. Inflammation of alveolar spaces caused by infection

    or aspiration is called _____.
37. A common respiratory problem characterized by a voluntary increase in the rate and volume of breathing often accompanied by anxiety is

    termed _____ _____.
38. The mnemonic used to assess the mental status of a

    patient is _____.
39. The rate of artificial ventilation for a nonbreathing

    adult is _____.

40. The rate of artificial ventilation for a nonbreathing child (age 1-8 years) is _____.

41. The rate of artificial ventilation for a nonbreathing infant (age <1 year) is _____.

SHORT ANSWER

Questions 42-47. List the six key questions to ask the patient with a respiratory emergency.

42. _____
    _____

43. _____
    _____

44. _____
    _____

45. _____
    _____

46. _____
    _____

47. _____
    _____

CASE SCENARIOS

Questions 48 to 51 refer to the following scenario.
You respond to a call at a local elementary school, where you find a 7-year-old girl in the nurse's office. The school nurse tells you that the girl has a history of asthma and came into the office complaining of difficulty breathing while participating in her gym class. Your evaluation reveals a patient in severe respiratory distress, with a respiratory rate of 36 breaths/min and labored, heart rate of 132 beats/min, and blood pressure of 84/60 mm Hg.

48. Your evaluation of this patient's blood pressure reveals a reading that:
    a. Is very low for this patient.
    b. Is very high for this patient.
    c. Should decrease significantly once the patient's respiratory distress is relieved.
    d. Is in the normal range for this patient.

49. If this patient were having an asthma attack, you would generally expect that auscultation of the lungs would reveal:
    a. Absent breath sounds on one side
    b. Full and clear bilateral breath sounds
    c. Wheezes
    d. Crackles (rales)

50. During transport to the hospital, you administer oxygen to the patient by nonrebreather mask. The patient's respiratory rate decreases from 36 to 10 breaths/min. The patient still appears to be in severe respiratory distress. This decrease in respiratory rate is:
    a. An ominous sign that respiratory failure/arrest may be imminent.
    b. A sign of oxygen toxicity.
    c. An indication that the patient's airway has become obstructed.
    d. A good sign that the patient is improving.

51. You are approximately 3 minutes from the hospital when the patient stops breathing, but still has a pulse at a rate of 124 beats/min. You should:
    a. Begin positive-pressure ventilation at a rate of 10 times per minute until the pop-off valve on the bag-mask is triggered.
    b. Begin positive-pressure ventilation at a rate of 20 times per minute until the pop-off valve on the bag-mask is triggered.
    c. Begin positive-pressure ventilation at a rate of 10 times per minute until you see chest rise.
    d. Begin positive-pressure ventilation at a rate of 20 times per minute until you see chest rise.

Questions 52 to 54 refer to the following scenario.
You respond to a call and find a 63-year-old man in the kitchen in severe respiratory distress. The patient is breathing through pursed lips, and his skin appears pink. The patient tells you that he has a history of emphysema and that his breathing difficulty has been worsening for the past 6 hours. The patient's pulse is 104 beats/min, blood pressure 142/86 mm Hg, and respiratory rate 24 breaths/min. The patient tells you that he normally smokes three packs of cigarettes a day, but today he has only smoked two packs because of his trouble breathing.

52. The type of disease affecting this patient is considered to be:
    a. A type of chronic obstructive pulmonary disease
    b. A severe form of pneumonia
    c. Caused by coronary artery disease
    d. One that can be cured with proper medical care

53. As part of treatment of this patient, you:
    a. Withhold any supplemental oxygen because of the patient's medical history.
    b. Administer oxygen by a nasal cannula at 2 L/min.
    c. Administer oxygen by a nonrebreather mask.
    d. Begin positive-pressure ventilations.

54. As you further examine the patient, you observe that he can be described as having a "barrel chest" appearance. This is caused by:
    a. Continuous use of supplemental oxygen in the home
    b. Excessive smoking
    c. Excessive alcohol consumption
    d. Air trapping in the lungs

69

Questions 55 and 56 refer to the following scenario.
You are called to the scene of the local community college and encounter a 20-year-old woman who is breathing very rapidly. The patient's friends tell you that the patient has anxiety attacks and became very nervous after the final examination scores were posted in her class. The patient is alert and complains only of difficulty breathing associated with tingling in the mouth and fingers. Vital signs are pulse of 104 beats/min and regular, blood pressure of 116/72 mm Hg, and respiratory rate of 28 breaths/min; the patient has full, clear bilateral breath sounds. The patient tells you that she does not take any medications, is not allergic to anything, and only has a history of anxiety attacks.

55. Your treatment for this patient includes:
    a. Having the patient breathe in and out with a paper bag over her mouth and nose.
    b. Having the patient hold her breath in an attempt to "break" the attack.
    c. Administering oxygen by a nonrebreather oxygen mask.
    d. Performing positive-pressure ventilations.

56. You have been treating the patient for the past 10 minutes while you transport her to the hospital. Your estimated arrival time at the hospital is 5 minutes. You reevaluate the patient and now find that her vital signs are pulse 92 beats/min and regular, blood pressure 112/68 mm Hg, and respiratory rate 16 breaths/min; the patient still has full, clear bilateral breath sounds. The change in this patient's respiratory rate is:
    a. An ominous sign of impending respiratory failure/arrest.
    b. A good indication that the patient is responding appropriately to treatment.
    c. An indication of oxygen toxicity.
    d. An indication that that the patient's underlying medical problem may be a pneumothorax.

57. Put the following steps for administering a medication through a nebulizer in proper sequential order.

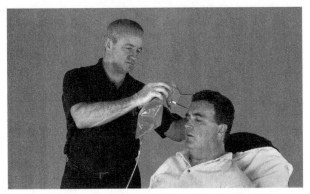

a. Remove the oxygen delivery device from the patient.

b. Monitor patient and medication. Have the patient continue to breathe through the nebulizer until the medication is depleted, about 5 to 15 minutes.

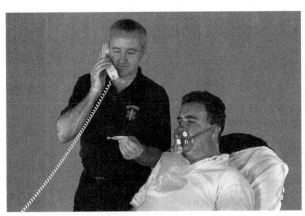

c. Check for allergies, and obtain an order from medical direction, either online or offline.

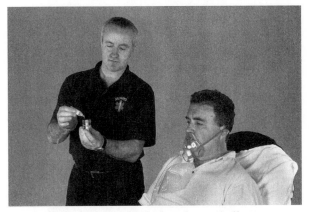

d. Pour contents of unit dose into nebulizer chamber.

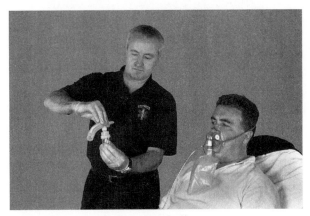

e. Screw top back onto nebulizer.

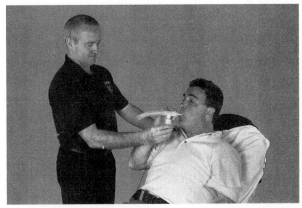

f. In the adult patient, attach nebulizer oxygen tubing to regulator and set at 6 L/min of flow. Instruct patient to breathe in and out through nebulizer mouthpiece. In a young child, hold the mouthpiece at the opening of the patient's mouth, and instruct the child to inhale normally (blow-by technique).

71

Chapter **11 Respiratory Emergencies**

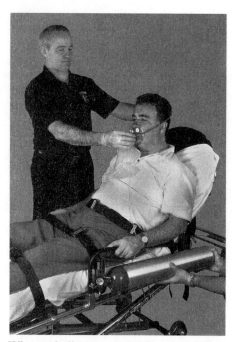

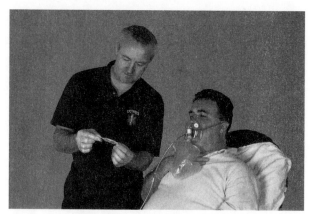

h. Check the medication *three times* for the following: correct medication, correct dose, correct patient, expiration date, loss of clarity or discoloration, and particulate matter.
- First check: When first selecting medication
- Second check: After pouring medication into nebulizer
- Third check: Before administering medication to the patient

g. When nebulizer treatment is completed, reattach oxygen administration device. Reevaluate the patient, and if appropriate, contact medical direction for additional treatment.

Correct Order

1. _____
2. _____
3. _____
4. _____
5. _____
6. _____
7. _____
8. _____

12 Cardiovascular Emergencies

MULTIPLE CHOICE

1. The protein responsible for the transport of oxygen and carbon dioxide is called:
   a. Protoplasm
   b. Platelets
   c. Plasma
   d. Hemoglobin
2. The cellular portions of the blood that are responsible for combating infection are the:
   a. Platelets
   b. Red blood cells
   c. White blood cells
   d. Hemoglobin
3. The portion of the heart that pumps blood to the body (systemic circulation) is called the:
   a. Left atrium
   b. Right atrium
   c. Left ventricle
   d. Right ventricle
4. The valve that directs blood into the pulmonary artery during systole and prevents backflow into the right ventricle during diastole is called the:
   a. Aortic valve
   b. Pulmonary semilunar valve
   c. Tricuspid valve
   d. Mitral valve
5. The portion of the conduction system that is the primary pacemaker of the heart is called the:
   a. Sinoatrial node
   b. Purkinje fiber
   c. Atrioventricular node
   d. Bundle of His
6. The amount of blood ejected from the heart with each contraction is called the:
   a. Cardiac output
   b. Tidal volume
   c. Cardiac reserve
   d. Stroke volume
7. The femoral, popliteal, and dorsalis pedis arteries are all located in the:
   a. Head
   b. Lower extremities
   c. Upper extremities
   d. Trunk
8. Which phase of the cardiac cycle does the diastolic pressure best reflect?
   a. Contraction
   b. Relaxation
   c. Intermediate period
   d. Rapid firing

9. The upper receiving chambers of the heart are called the:
   a. Ventricles
   b. Septa
   c. Atria
   d. Pleura
10. The circulation originating from the left side of the heart is the:
    a. Pulmonary circulation
    b. Systemic circulation
    c. Arterial circulation
    d. Venous circulation
11. The circulation originating from the right side of the heart is the:
    a. Pulmonary circulation
    b. Systemic circulation
    c. Arterial circulation
    d. Venous circulation
12. The valves that control flow from the atria to the ventricles are the:
    a. Semilunar valves
    b. Atrioventricular valves
    c. Atrial valves
    d. Ventricular valves
13. Gas exchange occurs in which of the following vessels?
    a. Arteries
    b. Veins
    c. Capillaries
    d. Venules
14. Shock that occurs from a myocardial infarction (heart attack) is called:
    a. Cardiogenic shock
    b. Distributive shock
    c. Obstructive shock
    d. Hypovolemic shock
15. The progressive narrowing of vessels because of plaque formation on the innermost lining best describes:
    a. Angioedema
    b. Arteriosclerosis
    c. Angina pectoris
    d. Ischemia
16. A patient who is demonstrating generalized signs of hypoxia (i.e., cyanosis or altered mental state) and severe chest pain should receive oxygen by a:
    a. Nasal cannula
    b. Nonrebreather mask
    c. Simple face mask
    d. Venturi mask

Chapter **12** **Cardiovascular Emergencies**

17. Which of the following is routinely used to self-administer nitroglycerin?
    a. Subcutaneous injection
    b. Intramuscular injection
    c. Ingest solution
    d. Spray or tablet placed under tongue
18. An insufficient supply of blood through a vessel that results in oxygen deprivation to tissue best describes:
    a. Ischemia
    b. Hypoxia
    c. Anoxia
    d. Anemia
19. Blockage of a coronary artery resulting in death of heart tissue defines:
    a. Coronary insufficiency
    b. Myocardial infarction
    c. Angina pectoris
    d. Cardiac arrest
20. Nausea, vomiting, weakness, shortness of breath, palpitations, lightheadedness, sweating, dizziness, and loss of consciousness are all possible associated signs of:
    a. Cardiac arrest
    b. Angina pectoris
    c. Myocardial infarction
    d. Oxygen toxicity
21. Chest pain brought on by emotional or physical exertion and relieved by rest best describes:
    a. Pleuritic chest pain
    b. Angina pectoris
    c. Myocardial infarction
    d. Cardiogenic shock
22. The patient should be questioned about high blood pressure, heart disease, chronic obstructive pulmonary disease, and diabetes during the:
    a. Chief complaint
    b. History of present illness
    c. Medications and allergies history
    d. Past medical history
23. Nitroglycerin acts to relieve chest pain by which of the following mechanisms?
    a. Increases heart rate.
    b. Increases the force of contraction.
    c. Causes vasodilation.
    d. Increases blood pressure.
24. Which of the following terms best describes the classic pain of cardiovascular disease, such as angina or myocardial infarction?
    a. Sharp
    b. Crushing
    c. Pleuritic
    d. Stabbing
25. The pulse of a patient having a myocardial infarction is usually:
    a. Rapid
    b. Almost any variation
    c. Slow
    d. Irregular

26. A common reaction to serious illness, including myocardial infarction, that often causes the patient to *not* seek help is referred to as:
    a. Rationalization
    b. Denial
    c. Confabulation
    d Anxiety syndrome
27. Myocardial infarction patients who have shortness of breath usually prefer to be placed in what position?
    a. Sitting
    b. Supine
    c. Prone
    d. Lateral recumbent
28. Patients who take nitroglycerin may have which of the following side effects?
    a. Hives
    b. Arrhythmias
    c. Headache
    d. Edema
29. The two most important factors in the treatment of prehospital cardiac arrest are cardiopulmonary resuscitation (CPR) and:
    a. Defibrillation
    b. Drug therapy
    c. Intubation
    d. Catheterization
30. A 55-year-old man experienced severe, pressurelike chest pain for 3 minutes after walking up two flights of stairs. He is alert, and his skin is pale, cool, and sweaty. His vital signs are pulse 100 beats/min and regular, respirations 20 breaths/min and normal, and blood pressure 160/90 mm Hg. In which position should this patient be placed?
    a. Supine
    b. Lateral recumbent
    c. Prone
    d. A position of comfort
31. Which of the following is the first and most important treatment provided by the EMT for the patient with chest pain?
    a. Administering oxygen.
    b. Rapidly transporting to the hospital.
    c. Attaching the automated external defibrillator (AED).
    d. Assisting the patient in the administration of nitroglycerin.
32. A patient tells you that he has angina pectoris but has *not* taken his prescribed nitroglycerin tablets today. How should you assist him in administration of nitroglycerin?
    a. Have him swallow 1 tablet and drink 10 mL of water.
    b. Do not administer the tablet; 3 minutes after the start of pain is too late to take the tablet.
    c. Place 1 tablet under the tongue, with no water.
    d. Have him swallow 3 tablets and drink 10 mL of water.

Chapter **12** **Cardiovascular Emergencies**

33. What is the maximum number of nitroglycerin tablets that a patient can receive for an angina attack?
    a. 1
    b. 2
    c. 3
    d. 4

34. A patient who usually takes 1 nitroglycerin tablet to relieve chest pain takes 3 tablets today, and his chest pain decreases slightly. He does not want to go to the hospital but must be urged to do so because of:
    a. Malignant hypertension
    b. Poor brain perfusion
    c. Sweaty skin
    d. Changing pattern of disease

35. If an angina patient's chest pain continues for 20 minutes, which of the following conditions should you suspect?
    a. Angina pectoris
    b. Myocardial infarction
    c. Cardiogenic shock
    d. Heart failure

36. You find a 62-year-old woman with nausea, dizziness, and pale sweaty skin complaining of crushing chest pain for 1 hour radiating to her left arm; her pulse is 110 beats/min and very irregular, blood pressure 160/100 mm Hg, and respirations 28 breaths/min and slightly labored. You suspect:
    a. Muscle strain
    b. Congestive heart failure
    c. Cardiogenic shock
    d. Acute coronary syndromes

37. What is the most common cause of death from myocardial infarction?
    a. Shock
    b. Ventricular fibrillation
    c. Pulmonary edema
    d. Respiratory failure

38. What is the most common cause of myocardial infarction?
    a. Poor circulation caused by arrhythmias
    b. Blockage of a coronary artery
    c. Overstretching of the ventricle
    d. Bleeding into the arterial wall

39. Besides the prompt application of CPR, which variable will most affect the survival of a cardiac arrest patient?
    a. Extent of the heart attack
    b. Time to defibrillation
    c. Ventilation device used during CPR
    d. Compression rate

40. The chaotic electrical rhythm that causes sudden clinical death in most cardiac arrest patients is called:
    a. Ventricular asystole
    b. Ventricular fibrillation
    c. Ventricular tachycardia
    d. Ventricular standstill

41. The origin of prehospital defibrillation dates back to the:
    a. 1940s
    b. 1950s
    c. 1960s
    d. 1970s

42. Defibrillation pads are positioned just below the right clavicle on the right sternal border and:
    a. Just below the left clavicle
    b. Directly over the midsternum
    c. Just left of the left nipple, midaxillary line
    d. Just above the left nipple, midclavicular line

43. When treating a patient in cardiac arrest, the AED is applied and shocks the patient once. After the shock, the appropriate action is to:
    a. Perform CPR immediately.
    b. Perform a precordial thump to stimulate the heart.
    c. Press "analyze" and shock as indicated.
    d. Check for signs of circulation; if none, perform CPR for 2 minutes and reanalyze.

44. While en route to the hospital, a patient becomes unconscious and pulseless. While your partner prepares the AED, what immediate action should you take?
    a. Administer oxygen by nonrebreather mask.
    b. Perform CPR.
    c. Give nitroglycerin.
    d. Monitor pulse and breathing.

45. To apply an AED, a patient must be:
    a. Having a confirmed heart attack
    b. Unconscious and pulseless
    c. At least 20 years old
    d. In the prone position

46. AEDs are useful to:
    a. Asystole and bradyarrhythmias
    b. Pulseless electrical activity
    c. Ventricular fibrillation and ventricular tachycardia
    d. Atrial fibrillation and atrial tachycardia

47. Which of the following patients should have an AED attached?
    a. 6-year-old boy having a seizure
    b. 46-year-old man complaining of chest pain
    c. Pulseless 25-year-old woman
    d. 58-year-old man complaining of fluttering in chest

48. If you apply the AED and it has advised "no shock," you should:
    a. Perform CPR for 2 minutes and reanalyze.
    b. Continue analyzing for 1 hour until it advises you to shock.
    c. Always pronounce the patient dead in the field.
    d. Check the machine for the correct operation.

Chapter **12 Cardiovascular Emergencies**

49. The act of applying an AED, analyzing, and defibrillating in a moving ambulance:
   a. Is not appropriate because it may shock a normal rhythm.
   b. Is important to reduce time to defibrillation.
   c. Should be done if the patient is pulseless.
   d. Helps facilitate rapid analysis of the rhythm.
50. The major advantage of an AED over a manual defibrillator is the ability to:
   a. Provide defibrillation with little or no operator knowledge of ECG.
   b. Deliver higher energy with the use of pads.
   c. Provide voice prompts that calm the operator during the emergency.
   d. Shock asystole, which a manual defibrillator will not shock.
51. After shocking a patient back to a normal rhythm, the patient becomes pulseless during transport to the hospital. You should:
   a. Stop the vehicle, analyze, and shock if advised.
   b. Continue CPR until you arrive at the hospital.
   c. Continue driving, and analyze and shock while en route.
   d. Administer a precordial thump, and start CPR.
52. When a patient remains in cardiac arrest, the primary reason for *not* checking a pulse after each shock with an AED is:
   a. The machine will tell you if a pulse is present.
   b. To minimize the disruption of performing CPR compressions.
   c. Pulses are irrelevant with AEDs.
   d. To expedite transport of the patient to the hospital.
53. The national organization that designs training programs and establishes guidelines for defibrillator use is the:
   a. American Board of EMTs
   b. American College of Cardiology
   c. American Heart Association
   d. American Association of Emergency Physicians
54. The best method for ensuring competency with AEDs is:
   a. Frequent hands-on practice
   b. Written reviews
   c. Device maintenance
   d. Mental drills
55. The review of events after AED use for a cardiac arrest patient is usually performed by:
   a. The EMT who managed the case
   b. Another EMT
   c. The medical director or designee
   d. The EMS administrator

56. Which statement best describes the relationship between cardiovascular compromise and cardiac arrest?
   a. All patients who have cardiovascular compromise will sustain a cardiac arrest.
   b. Cardiovascular compromise will rarely evolve into a cardiac arrest situation.
   c. Patients who sustain cardiovascular compromise are at high risk of sudden cardiac arrest.
   d. Cardiac arrest usually occurs after several hours of cardiovascular compromise.
57. Patients with chest pain should be routinely attached to an AED.
   a. True
   b. False
58. If you are alone with a pulseless patient (witnessed arrest) and you have an AED, what action should you take first after determining breathlessness and pulselessness?
   a. Perform CPR for 1 minute.
   b. Attach the AED and begin operation.
   c. Perform CPR until helps arrives.
   d. Perform one shock and start CPR.
59. The normal dose of aspirin is:
   a. 81 to 160 mg
   b. 160 to 325 mg
   c. 250 to 500 mg
   d. 325 to 625 mg
60. Which of the following is the correct action when you have applied the AED pads to the hairy chest of a patient in cardiac arrest and are receiving a "check electrode" message from the AED?
   a. Discontinue use of the AED.
   b. Press down firmly on the AED pads.
   c. Use a separate adhesive to secure the pads firmly.
   d. Hold the pads on the chest wall while the AED analyzes.
61. Which of the following is the correct action with a patient who has a transdermal medication patch on the chest where you are about to attach an AED pad?
   a. Use the AED as normal; the medication patch, even if under the AED pad, will not interfere with the AED's operation.
   b. Do not use the AED; there is a risk of explosion if the medication patch contains nitroglycerin.
   c. Remove the medication patch, and wipe the area clean; then use the AED as normal.
   d. Remove the medication patch, and dilute the area with vinegar before using the AED.

MATCHING

Questions 62-66. Match the type of heart failure in column B with the signs and symptoms in column A.

Column A
62. _____ Rales
63. _____ Ankle edema
64. _____ Frothy sputum
65. _____ Distended neck veins
66. _____ Ascites

Column B
a. Right-sided heart failure
b. Left-sided heart failure

SHORT ANSWER

Questions 67-69. List three contraindications to the administration of aspirin:

67. _____

_____

68. _____

_____

69. _____

_____

Questions 70-75. List the six key questions that you should ask the patient with a cardiac emergency.

70. _____

_____

71. _____

_____

72. _____

_____

73. _____

_____

74. _____

_____

75. _____

_____

Questions 76-79. List the four links in the chain of survival.

76. _____

_____

77. _____

_____

78. _____

_____

79. _____

_____

Questions 80-88. List nine common associated complaints that may be present in the patient with chest pain.

80. _____

_____

81. _____

_____

82. _____

_____

83. _____

_____

84. _____

_____

85. _____

_____

86. _____

_____

87. _____

_____

88. _____

_____

CASE SCENARIOS

Questions 89 to 92 refer to the following scenario.
You respond to a call at the local gym and encounter a 50-year-old man on the floor next to an exercise bicycle. Bystanders tell you that the patient got off the cycle, sat on the floor, and then collapsed. His blood pressure is 72/40 mm Hg, heart rate 30 beats/min, and respiratory rate 4 breaths/min.

89. Your initial management for this patient includes:
   a. Connecting the AED to the patient and analyzing the patient's heart rhythm.
   b. Positioning the patient supine with his head elevated and providing positive-pressure ventilations.
   c. Positioning the patient supine with his legs elevated and providing positive-pressure ventilations.
   d. Positioning the patient supine with his legs elevated and delivering supplemental oxygen with a nonrebreather mask.

77

90. You are en route to the hospital when you no longer feel the patient's pulse and respirations cease. Your estimated drive time to the hospital is 20 minutes. You should:
    a. Have your partner continue driving to the hospital while you connect the AED and analyze the patient's heart rhythm.
    b. Have your partner pull over to the side of the road, and then connect the AED and analyze the patient's heart rhythm.
    c. Begin and continue CPR until you reach the hospital.
    d. Perform CPR for 5 minutes, and if the patient is still in cardiac arrest, connect the AED and analyze the patient's heart rhythm.

91. Approximately 5 minutes before arriving at the hospital, the patient has a return of spontaneous circulation. You reevaluate the patient, and his heart rate is 72 beats/min, blood pressure 142/76 mm Hg, and respiration 14 breaths/min and adequate. You should:
    a. Continue positive-pressure ventilations.
    b. Administer oxygen at 2 to 3 L/min with a nasal cannula.
    c. Open the airway with the head-tilt/chin-lift method; no supplemental oxygen is required.
    d. Administer oxygen with a nonrebreather mask.

92. You are now 2 minutes from the hospital when the patient begins to vomit. The best position to place this patient in is:
    a. Supine
    b. Prone
    c. Left lateral recumbent
    d. Supine with legs elevated

Questions 93 to 95 refer to the following scenario.
Your EMS unit is on standby at the high school football game. You are summoned to the sidelines to treat a 42-year-old coach who became very dizzy. The patient informs you that he has a cardiac history and sometimes takes nitroglycerin. He has his prescribed nitroglycerin pills, which have not expired. Vital signs are pulse 86 beats/min and regular but weak, blood pressure 120/60 mm Hg, and respiratory rate 20 breaths/min and normal. Your drive time to the hospital is approximately 12 minutes.

93. You continue to evaluate your patient and begin to ask questions specific to the patient's chief complaint. You would ask the patient:
    a. Do you have any chest pain or chest discomfort?
    b. Do you have any sharp chest pain?
    c. Do you have any pressure in your chest?
    d. Do you have a squeezing sensation in your chest?

94. Your treatment for this patient includes:
    a. Oxygen by nonrebreather mask and assisting the patient in taking 1 nitroglycerin tablet.
    b. Oxygen by nonrebreather mask and connecting the AED to the patient.
    c. Oxygen by nonrebreather mask and rapid transport.
    d. Assisting the patient in taking 1 nitroglycerin tablet.

95. While placing the patient on your ambulance stretcher, the patient appears to have seizurelike activity that lasts for approximately 30 seconds. You reevaluate your patient and determine that he is now in cardiac arrest. You should:
    a. Begin CPR and transport the patient to the hospital.
    b. Withhold CPR because CPR is not indicated in a patient who has had a seizure.
    c. Withhold CPR until an AED is available.
    d. Begin CPR and connect the AED to the patient as soon as possible.

96. Put the following steps in performing one-person cardiopulmonary resuscitation in proper sequential order.

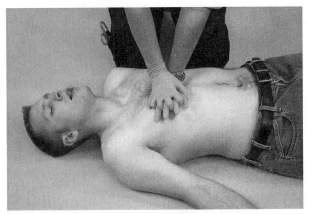

a. Perform external chest compressions at a rate of 100 compressions per minute with a compression/ventilation ratio of 30:2. Depress the chest 1½ to 2 inches with each compression. Perform 5 complete cycles of 30 compressions and 2 ventilations. Reevaluate after 5 cycles of compressions and ventilations.

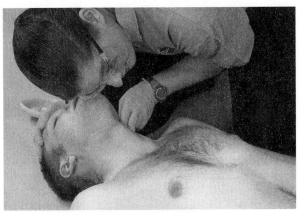

c. Check for a carotid pulse (no more than 10 and no less than 5 seconds). If there is no pulse, begin chest compressions.

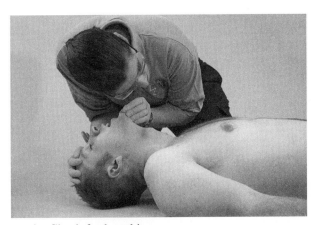

b. Check for breathing.

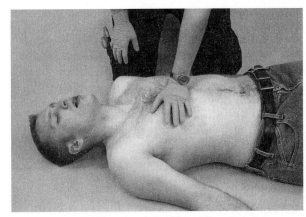

d. Locate proper hand position. Place hand at midnipple line.

Chapter **12** **Cardiovascular Emergencies**

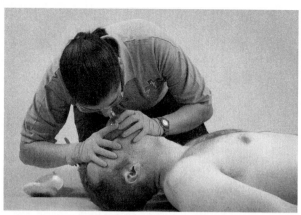

e. If not breathing, begin rescue breathing with 2 initial breaths and 1 breath every 5 to 6 seconds.

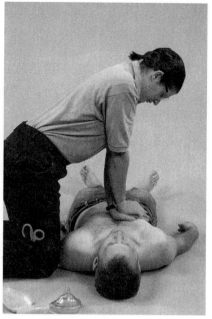

g. Depress the chest 1½ to 2 inches with each compression. Perform 5 complete cycles of 30 compressions and 2 ventilations. Reevaluate after 5 cycles of compressions and ventilations.

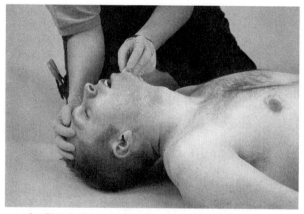

f. Check for unresponsiveness. Open the airway with the head-tilt/chin-lift or jaw thrust maneuver.

Correct Order

1. _____

2. _____

3. _____

4. _____

5. _____

6. _____

7. _____

13 Altered Mental Status

MULTIPLE CHOICE

1. Stored forms of glucose can be released between meals. This process is initiated by the hormone:
   a. LDH
   b. Progesterone
   c. Glycogen
   d. Glucagon

2. Patients with a severe or absolute lack of insulin have:
   a. Non-insulin-dependent diabetes
   b. Insulin-dependent diabetes
   c. Glucose-dependent diabetes
   d. Glycogen-dependent diabetes

3. Non-insulin-dependent diabetic patients usually take medication that stimulates the pancreas to produce:
   a. Glucose
   b. Fructose
   c. Glycogen
   d. Insulin

4. Diabetes is a disease that results from an inadequate secretion of the hormone:
   a. Insulin
   b. Epinephrine
   c. Glucagon
   d. Progesterone

5. Insulin helps regulate the use and storage of:
   a. Ketones
   b. Isotones
   c. Glucose
   d. Epinephrine

6. What does the brain primarily rely on for nourishment?
   a. Insulin
   b. Glycogen
   c. Glucose
   d. Glucagon

7. Insulin is produced within specialized cells in the:
   a. Liver
   b. Spleen
   c. Pancreas
   d. Adrenal gland

8. Some glucose is stored in the liver and muscle as a larger molecule called:
   a. Glucagon
   b. Glycogen
   c. Fructose
   d. Insulin

9. A diabetic emergency that develops from a lack of insulin and elevated blood glucose causing dehydration and acidosis is:
   a. Diabetic encephalopathy
   b. Diabetic ketoacidosis
   c. Diabetic syndrome
   d. Insulin shock

10. The most common and treatable diabetic problem encountered in prehospital care that results from a lack of available sugar in the blood is:
    a. Diabetic coma
    b. Hypoglycemia
    c. Hyperosmolar coma
    d. Diabetic encephalopathy

11. Signs of hypoglycemia may include hunger, nausea, weakness, and:
    a. Dry mouth
    b. Bizarre behavior
    c. Slow pulse
    d. Hypotension

12. A drug that is given intramuscularly for hypoglycemia and that may be carried at times by the patient is:
    a. Glucose
    b. Glucagon
    c. Glycogen
    d. Insulin

13. Before giving a conscious diabetic patient an oral glucose gel, you should:
    a. Check for a gag reflex.
    b. Take two sets of vital signs.
    c. Lay the patient supine.
    d. Give the patient two glasses of water.

14. Which of the following is a trade name for oral glucose:
    a. Glucometer
    b. Glucagon
    c. Glutose
    d. Glugel

15. If a situation is unclear regarding the history and physical assessment of a suspected diabetic patient, you should:
    a. Disregard the history and proceed with the treatment.
    b. Discuss the situation with your partner and proceed with the treatment.
    c. Consult with medical direction before treatment.
    d. Not be concerned; the history and physical assessment are not important for these patients.

MATCHING

Questions 16-23. Match the signs and symptoms in column A with the diabetic emergency in column B.

Column A   **Column B**
16. _____ Increased thirst   a. Hypoglycemia
17. _____ Sweaty skin   b. Diabetic ketoacidosis
18. _____ Pale skin
19. _____ Increased urination
20. _____ Salivation
21. _____ Combative behavior
22. _____ Acetone and deep
          respiration
23. _____ Fruity breath odor

FILL IN THE BLANK

Questions 24-28. Write a word in the blank to complete the sentence.

24. A reversible episode of focal neurologic dysfunction that typically lasts a few minutes to a few hours and resolves within 24 hours is called

    a(n) _____ _____ _____.

25. _____ is the most common cause of intracerebral hemorrhage.

26. A stroke is also referred to as a(n) _____
    _____.

27. A blood clot that moves in the bloodstream and migrates to the brain causing a stroke is referred to

    as a(n) _____.

28. A clot that develops within a brain artery itself is

    referred to as a(n) _____.

SHORT ANSWER

Questions 29-38. List 10 possible causes of a seizure.

29. _____
    _____

30. _____
    _____

31. _____
    _____

32. _____
    _____

33. _____
    _____

34. _____

35. _____
    _____

36. _____
    _____

37. _____
    _____

38. _____
    _____

TRUE/FALSE

39. _____ Hemorrhagic strokes are the most common type of stroke.
40. _____ Hypotension is typically caused by a stroke.
41. _____ The use of a prehospital stroke scale is useful to predict the patient's neurologic outcome.
42. _____ The presence of an acute stroke is an indication for rapid transport.
43. _____ Patients with a hemorrhagic stroke can often be treated with "clot busting" medications if they arrive at the hospital within a few hours of symptom onset.
44. _____ A history of transient ischemic attacks is a significant indicator of stroke risk.
45. _____ Stroke is the leading cause of death in the United States in adults.

CASE SCENARIOS

Questions 46 to 49 are based on the following scenario.

You respond to a local nursing home for an 82-year-old woman found in her bed and unresponsive to verbal or painful stimuli. The nurse's aide informs you that the patient is in the nursing home for rehabilitation after surgery to replace her left hip. Normally the patient is alert and oriented and can ambulate with a walker. It is now 1400 hours. The patient has a history of "irregular" heartbeats but is not taking any medications. The patient was last seen awake and alert at approximately 1000 hours. The patient's vital signs are pulse of 88 beats/min and irregular, blood pressure of 156/92 mm Hg, and respiratory rate of 16 breaths/min and adequate.

46. The best term to describe this patient's altered mental state is:
    a. Lethargy
    b. Stupor
    c. Semicoma
    d. Coma
47. Based on the patient's clinical presentation, you suspect that the patient is experiencing:
    a. An acute cardiac condition
    b. A drug overdose
    c. Hypoglycemia
    d. A stroke

48. As you further evaluate the patient, you determine that she does not open her eyes, does not make any verbal sounds, and does not move despite painful stimuli. What would this patient's score be on the Glasgow Coma Scale?
    a. 0
    b. 3
    c. 10
    d. 15
49. Prehospital management of this patient includes:
    a. Administration of oral glucose and transport to the nearest hospital.
    b. Airway management and rapid transport to the appropriate hospital.
    c. Contact with poison control for permission to administer a cathartic.
    d. Connecting the patient to an AED to be prepared if she goes into cardiac arrest.

Questions 50 to 52 refer to the following scenario.
You respond to a business office and find a 37-year-old woman lying on the floor who has a depressed level of consciousness and is confused. Co-workers tell you that the patient appeared to have a seizure. You ask them exactly what the patient was exhibiting during the seizure, and they describe intermittent contractions and relaxations of the muscles, which "looked like jerking movements."

50. The activity that is described to you by the co-workers is termed the:
    a. Tonic phase of a seizure
    b. Clonic phase of a seizure
    c. Postictal period
    d. Aura
51. While you continue to examine the patient, she slowly begins to awake but still appears to be confused. This stage of a seizure is called the:
    a. Tonic phase
    b. Clonic phase
    c. Postictal period
    d. Aura
52. While you begin transport of the patient to the ambulance, she begins to exhibit signs of a grand mal seizure. The seizure continues as you prepare the patient for transport. If the seizure were to continue for more than 5 minutes, it would be termed:
    a. A petit mal seizure
    b. Irreversible brain damage
    c. Status epilepticus
    d. Convulsions

CROSSWORD PUZZLE

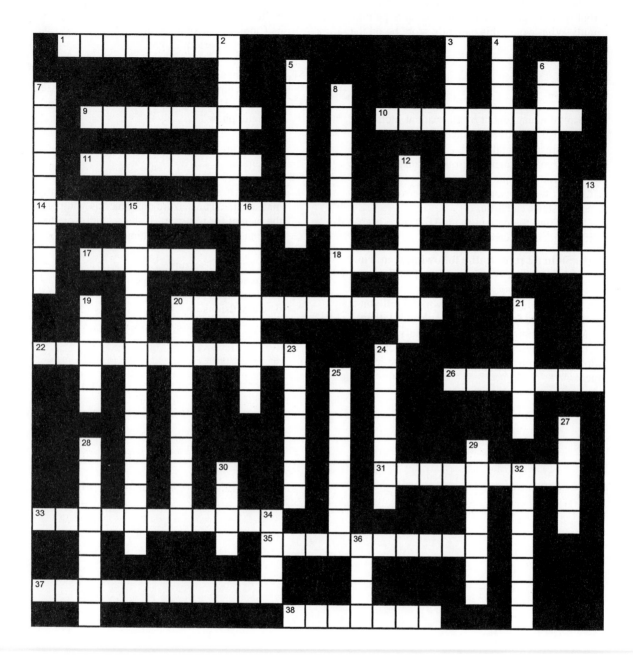

Chapter **13** **Altered Mental Status**

Across

1. Disease caused by an inadequate secretion of insulin
9. Bluish discoloration of mucous membranes or skin
10. The area that is the center for receiving and processing visual stimuli
11. Medication that converts glycogen back to glucose
14. "Stroke"
17. Seizure phase characterized by intermittent contractions and relaxations of the skeletal muscles resulting in rapid, jerky movements
18. High body temperature
20. Glucose deprivation
22. On finding a patient with an alteration in mental status, the EMT must first assess the adequacy of _____.
26. Bluish skin color is a sign of _____.
31. A patient who is easily aroused but drifts into a sleepy state without continued stimulation
33. Low body temperature
35. Damage to one side of the brain shows examination findings that are one sided or _____.
37. Scale used to measure a patient's mental status
38. Hormone that regulates the utilization and storage of glucose

Down

2. A condition marked by lack of awareness of the environment from which the patient may be aroused
3. _____ odor on the breath may be a sign of diabetic ketoacidosis.
4. The cerebrum is divided down the middle into right and left halves called _____.
5. The largest and most superior portion of the brain
6. The lower part of the brain
7. Final phase of a seizure with depressed level of consciousness and confusion
8. Symptoms for which no cause can be found
12. Stroke that occurs as the result of an occluded blood vessel supplying the brain
13. Toxemia of pregnancy—a potential for seizures
15. If the brain is deprived of oxygen, _____ _____ can occur in 4 to 6 minutes.
16. A patient who can be aroused but does not reach a normal level of consciousness and function
19. Phase of seizure with sustained contraction of all voluntary muscles
20. Warm, hot, dry skin suggests _____.
21. Third leading cause of death in the United States
23. Temporary alteration in behavior caused by abnormal electrical activity in the brain
24. Seizure in a child precipitated by a high fever and infection
25. A generalized seizure affecting the entire body
27. Seizures that may affect only a portion of the body or manifest as an alteration in consciousness
28. The area of the brain that receives smell and hearing signals
29. Artery that joins the carotids in the center of the brain
30. A patient in a _____ has no responsiveness to external stimuli.
32. A carbohydrate used by the cells for energy
34. Sensations or motor events that may warn the patient of an oncoming seizure
36. The patient's ability to respond to stimuli is measured using this mnemonic.

14 Allergies

MULTIPLE CHOICE

1. Anaphylaxis is a serious allergic reaction after patients come into contact with substances called _____ to which they have been previously sensitized.
   a. Antigens
   b. Antibodies
   c. Histamines
   d. Antihistamines

2. A substance that is released from cells during an anaphylactic reaction that can trigger blood vessels to dilate and capillaries to leak is called:
   a. An antigen
   b. An endorphin
   c. Histamine
   d. Adrenaline

3. Which of the following is a common agent for producing an anaphylactic reaction?
   a. Vegetables
   b. Shellfish
   c. Milk
   d. Fruit

4. Some anaphylactic patients may carry a kit that contains antihistamine agents and:
   a. Morphine
   b. Dilantin
   c. Epinephrine
   d. Phenobarbital

5. Anaphylactic reactions may present with raised, red patches of skin called:
   a. Erythema
   b. Purpura
   c. Urticaria (hives)
   d. Papules

6. The major lethal complications of anaphylaxis are circulatory collapse and:
   a. Arrhythmias
   b. Airway obstruction
   c. Urticaria (hives)
   d. Fluid overload

7. Epinephrine is usually administered to an adult through an autoinjector at a dose of:
   a. 0.3 mg
   b. 0.1 mg
   c. 0.2 mg
   d. 0.5 mg

8. Epinephrine is usually administered to a child through an autoinjector at a dose of:
   a. 0.15 mg
   b. 0.2 mg
   c. 0.25 mg
   d. 0.3 mg

9. The trade name for epinephrine is:
   a. Norepinephrine
   b. Acetylcholine
   c. Adrenalin
   d. Isoproterenol

10. What is the location for administration of an epinephrine autoinjector?
    a. Midlateral shoulder region
    b. Lower and outer quadrant of the buttocks
    c. Midlateral thigh region
    d. Mid-biceps muscle

11. Patients in anaphylaxis who are exhibiting signs of shock should be transported in what position?
    a. Left lateral recumbent
    b. Supine
    c. Supine with the legs elevated
    d. Supine with the head elevated

12. A patient with severe difficulty breathing, hives, and swelling of the mouth, neck, and tongue is likely experiencing:
    a. A minor allergic reaction
    b. Anaphylaxis
    c. Asthma or chronic obstructive pulmonary disease
    d. Epiglottitis

13. The EMT can treat complete airway obstruction from anaphylaxis with:
    a. Abdominal thrusts
    b. Extreme hyperextension
    c. Patient positioning
    d. Continued attempts at positive-pressure ventilation

MATCHING

Questions 14-17. Match the physiologic effects in column A to the signs and symptoms of anaphylaxis in column B.

Column A	Column B
14. _____ Constriction of bronchial smooth muscle	a. Hypotension
15. _____ Increased permeability of capillaries and fluid leakage	b. Swelling of the skin and stridor caused by obstruction
16. _____ Dilation of the arteries	c. Sneezing and nasal congestion
17. _____ Increased mucus secretions in the respiratory tree	d. Wheezing breath sounds

SHORT ANSWER

18. A patient with anaphylaxis shows some improvement after epinephrine administration but deteriorates during transport.

    You should _____.

Questions 19-28. List 10 of the 20 symptoms (patient complaints) that may be present in the anaphylactic patient.

19. _____

20. _____

21. _____

22. _____

23. _____

24. _____

25. _____

26. _____

27. _____

28. _____

Questions 29-38. List 10 of the 16 signs of anaphylaxis.

29. _____

30. _____

31. _____

32. _____

33. _____

34. _____

35. _____

36. _____

37. _____

38. _____

Questions 39-44. List the six key questions to ask the patient with an allergic reaction.

39. _____

40. _____

41. _____

42. _____

43. _____

44. _____

Questions 45-52. List the eight possible side effects that a patient may exhibit after the administration of epinephrine.

45. _____

46. _____

47. _____

48. _____

49. _____

50. _____

51. _____

    _____

52. _____

    _____

CASE SCENARIOS

Questions 53 to 56 refer to the following scenario.
You respond to a call at a ball field and encounter
a 23-year-old man in severe respiratory distress. His
friends tell you that the patient was stung by a bee on
his arm. Approximately 5 minutes after he was stung,
he began to have difficulty breathing, and a bystander
called 9-1-1. Your evaluation reveals a patient with
hives on his arm, torso, and chest. His lips appear to be
slightly swollen. The patient's blood pressure is
72/40 mm Hg, heart rate is 110 beats/min, and the
respiratory rate is 28 breaths/min. Your partner suggests
that you administer epinephrine to this patient.

53. Based on the physical examination of this
    patient, you:
    a. Withhold any epinephrine because of the
       patient's low blood pressure.
    b. Withhold any epinephrine because of the
       patient's age.
    c. Administer an EpiPen Jr. containing 0.15 mg of
       epinephrine.
    d. Administer an EpiPen containing 0.30 mg of
       epinephrine.

54. Your continued treatment of this patient includes:
    a. Remaining at the scene for 3 to 5 minutes to see
       if your initial treatment has any effect.
    b. Initiating humidified oxygen administration by
       a nasal cannula at 2 to 4 L/min.
    c. Initiating high-concentration oxygen administra-
       tion by a nonrebreather mask and rapid transport.
    d. Administering a Mark I kit.

55. If you administer epinephrine to this patient, you
    would expect that:
    a. The patient's heart rate will quickly decrease.
    b. The patient's heart rate will remain unchanged.
    c. The patient's heart rate will quickly increase.
    d. Any change in the patient's heart rate would
       depend on the specific cause of the allergic
       reaction.

56. During transport to the hospital, the patient's airway
    becomes totally obstructed by swelling of the neck
    and tongue. You should:
    a. Immediately perform abdominal thrusts.
    b. Immediately perform chest thrusts.
    c. Perform a jaw thrust and maintain oxygen
       delivery with a nonrebreather mask.
    d. Attempt to deliver positive-pressure ventilations.

Questions 57 and 58 refer to the following scenario.
You respond to a patient's home where you encounter
a 33-year-old woman who tells you that she is having a
severe allergic reaction to antibiotics that she just began
to take that morning. The patient has a history of
asthma but no other medical history or known
allergies. The patient is alert and has respiratory rate of
14 breaths/min, full clear bilateral breath sounds, pulse
of 92 beats/min and regular, and blood pressure of
124/72 mm Hg. The patient has no difficulty speaking
or swallowing. You notice a few hives on the patient's
upper torso.

57. Your immediate treatment for this patient includes:
    a. Administering an EpiPen Jr. containing
       0.15 mg of epinephrine.
    b. Administering an EpiPen containing 0.30 mg
       of epinephrine.
    c. Administering oxygen and transporting the
       patient to the hospital.
    d. Advising the patient that hospital evaluation is
       not needed and to call back if the symptoms
       progress.

58. Based on your evaluation of the patient,
    you suspect the patient may be having a(n):
    a. Minor allergic reaction
    b. Anaphylactic reaction
    c. Acute asthma attack
    d. Chronic obstructive pulmonary attack

15 Poisoning and Overdoses

1. A regional agency available for phone consultation in the event of a poisoning is called a(n):
   a. Toxicology center
   b. Abused substance center
   c. Poison control center
   d. Toxic ingestion center

2. The first priority in managing an unconscious suspected poison patient is to:
   a. Induce vomiting.
   b. Provide cardiorespiratory support.
   c. Hasten elimination of the poison.
   d. Keep the patient awake.

3. Three important questions regarding a poisoning incident are what was taken, how much was taken, and:
   a. Why it was taken.
   b. The age of the patient.
   c. Whether it was a suicide attempt.
   d. When it was taken.

4. Administering activated charcoal is designed to:
   a. Hasten elimination.
   b. Neutralize the poison.
   c. Prevent absorption by the body.
   d. Provide an antidote.

5. The primary antidote for a carbon monoxide poisoning is:
   a. Carbon dioxide
   b. Naloxone
   c. Oxygen
   d. EpiPen

6. The most common pupillary finding in opioid (narcotic) overdoses (e.g., heroin) is:
   a. Dilated
   b. Midpositional
   c. Unequal
   d. Pinpoint

7. The major complication of a narcotic overdose is:
   a. Arrhythmia
   b. Heart attack
   c. Respiratory arrest
   d. Bleeding

8. Fast heart rate, hypertension, chest pain, anxious behavior, delirium, and paranoia best describe an overdose of:
   a. Depressants
   b. Narcotics
   c. Sedative-hypnotics
   d. Stimulants

9. Alcohol is a central nervous system:
   a. Depressant
   b. Stimulant
   c. Hypnotic
   d. Hallucinogenic

10. A drug that may cause few or no symptoms immediately after taken in overdose, but that may lead to severe liver failure days later, is:
    a. Aspirin
    b. Diazepam (Valium)
    c. Amphetamine
    d. Acetaminophen

11. The first and most important step in the management of an inhalation poisoning is:
    a. Removal from the toxic environment
    b. Administration of oxygen
    c. Positive-pressure ventilation
    d. Cardiopulmonary resuscitation

12. Eyes that have been exposed to corrosive chemicals should be irrigated for a minimum of:
    a. 5 minutes
    b. 10 minutes
    c. 15 minutes
    d. 20 minutes

Questions 13-16. Match the type of poisoning in column A with the substance in column B.

Column A	Column B
13. _____ Ingestion	a. Carbon monoxide
14. _____ Inhalation	b. Organophosphates (insecticide) on skin
15. _____ Injection	c. Methanol
16. _____ Absorption	d. Scorpion sting

Questions 17-21. Match the diagnostic odor in column A with the possible substance in column B.

Column A	Column B
17. _____ Acetone (sweet, fruity)	a. Organophosphate
18. _____ Disinfectants	b. Methyl salicylate
19. _____ Eggs (rotten)	c. Ethanol, isopropyl alcohol, diabetic ketoacidosis
20. _____ Garlic	d. Hydrogen sulfide
21. _____ Wintergreen	e. Phenol, creosote

22. _____ _____ is the toxic substance contained in antifreeze.

23. _____ is the toxic substance found in automobile windshield-washing fluid.

24. The national toll-free number that should be accessed to contact the regional poison control

center is _____.

SHORT ANSWER

Questions 25-31. List the seven key questions to ask the patient with a poisoning/overdose.

25. _____

_____

26. _____

_____

27. _____

_____

28. _____

_____

29. _____

_____

30. _____

_____

31. _____

_____

CASE SCENARIOS

Questions 32 to 34 refer to the following scenario.
You respond to a call and find a 5-year-old girl who is suspected of having ingested 100 acetaminophen (Tylenol) tablets 10 minutes earlier. The mother shows you an empty bottle, but the child appears perfectly normal and has normal vital signs. The child is alert and oriented.

32. Normal vital signs in this type of overdose are:
    a. Possible but not likely.
    b. Likely in the first 24 hours.
    c. Possible only in the first few minutes.
    d. Highly unlikely after 5 minutes.

33. You contact medical direction for advice in treating this child. What first step would they likely advise under these circumstances?
    a. Give 15 mL of ipecac.
    b. Give several glasses of water.
    c. Give activated charcoal.
    d. Rapid transport only.

34. What would the likely treatment be for an ingestion of an alkali poison?
    a. Give 15 mL (1 tablespoon) of ipecac.
    b. Give one or two glasses of water or milk.
    c. Give activated charcoal.
    d. Rapid transport only.

Questions 35 to 38 refer to the following scenario.
You respond to a call and find a 50-year-old man locked in his garage with his car motor running. He is unresponsive and his skin is pink.

35. Your immediate action should be to:
    a. Open the garage door, turn off the car engine, and give high-concentration oxygen.
    b. Remove the patient from the garage and give high-concentration oxygen.
    c. Immediately transport the patient to the hospital to be intubated.
    d. Give humidified oxygen by nasal cannula and transport.

36. The pink skin color associated with carbon monoxide poisoning is from:
    a. Unsaturated hemoglobin
    b. Hemoglobin saturated with carbon dioxide
    c. Hemoglobin saturated with carbon monoxide
    d. Hemoglobin saturated with cyanide

37. Which of the following definitive treatments would be most helpful for treating a patient with carbon monoxide poisoning?
    a. Hyperbaric oxygen
    b. Intubation and ventilation
    c. Heart-lung machine
    d. Dialysis

38. Your immediate action is to:
    a. Open the airway and begin positive-pressure ventilation.
    b. Suction and administer oxygen by nasal cannula.
    c. Apply the pneumatic antishock garment.
    d. Induce vomiting.

Questions 39 to 41 refer to the following scenario.
You respond to an overdose and find a 22-year-old man with track marks on his arm who is unresponsive to painful stimuli. Physical examination reveals pinpoint pupils, and snoring is heard with each breath. His vital signs are respirations 10 breaths/min and shallow, pulse 62 beats/min and thready, and blood pressure 90/60 mm Hg.

39. Based on the signs and symptoms of the patient, you suspect:
    a. Amphetamine overdose
    b. Barbiturate overdose
    c. Opiate overdose
    d. Sedative-hypnotic overdose

40. You are en route to the hospital when the patient begins to vomit. Your immediate action is to:
    a. Perform the Heimlich maneuver.
    b. Place the patient prone and continue transport.
    c. Change your oxygen delivery mask to a nonrebreather oxygen mask.
    d. Use suction to clear the airway.

41. A patient has ingested a substance that might contraindicate the use of activated charcoal. What actions should you take?
    a. Contact medical direction for clarification.
    b. Proceed with administration of activated charcoal.
    c. Provide a lower dose of the activated charcoal.
    d. Do not administer the activated charcoal.

Questions 42 to 44 refer to the following scenario.
You respond to a suburban home where you find a neighbor frantically yelling that she can see her neighbors lying motionless on the floor in their living room. The neighbor tells you that she has been banging on the door, but no one is answering. The neighbor saw a fuel oil service truck leave the home about 3 hours ago.

42. Your first consideration in gaining access to these patients is to:
    a. Immediately break a window and enter the home to access the patients.
    b. Call for the specialized self-contained breathing apparatus team to access the house.
    c. Summon personnel to the scene with appropriate self-contained breathing devices.
    d. Enter the house while wearing an oxygen mask.

43. Once the patients are removed from the house, you begin your evaluation and determine that there are a total of three patients. All are responsive only to painful stimuli. One patient has a "pink" appearance; the other two patients appear pale. Based on the scene and your patient evaluations, you determine that the patients may have:
    a. Food poisoning
    b. Carbon monoxide poisoning
    c. An unknown drug overdose
    d. Smoke inhalation

44. The best treatment for these patients includes:
    a. Low-flow oxygen and transport to the local hospital 5 minutes away.
    b. High-flow oxygen and transport to the local hospital 5 minutes away.
    c. Low-flow oxygen and transport to the hyperbaric center 12 minutes away.
    d. High-flow oxygen and transport to the hyperbaric center 12 minutes away.

Questions 45 to 48 refer to the following scenario.
You respond to the local bus station and encounter an approximately 33-year-old man lying on the ground. The patient shows no visible trauma. Vital signs are pulse 92 beats/min and regular, respiratory rate 2 breaths/min, and blood pressure 142/76 mm Hg; the patient's pupils are very constricted. The patient's lips appear to be bluish in color.

45. Your immediate treatment for this patient is:
    a. Rapid transport.
    b. Administration of oxygen by a nonrebreather mask.
    c. Initiation of positive-pressure ventilations.
    d. Administration of a cathartic.

46. Based on your evaluation, you suspect:
    a. Carbon monoxide poisoning
    b. A narcotic overdose
    c. An acetaminophen overdose
    d. Anaphylactic shock

47. The bluish coloration in the patient's lips is caused by:
    a. Hemoglobin saturated with carbon monoxide
    b. Oxygen toxicity
    c. The patient hyperventilating
    d. Unsaturated hemoglobin

48. While en route to the hospital, you determine that the patient has gone into cardiac arrest (no pulse or respirations). Your estimated time of arrival at the hospital is 7 minutes. The use of the automated external defibrillator for this patient is:
    a. Contraindicated because of the cause of the cardiac arrest.
    b. Indicated and should be performed as soon as possible.
    c. Contraindicated because of the patient's age.
    d. Indicated only after there is no response to 5 minutes of cardiopulmonary resuscitation.

16 Environmental Emergencies

MULTIPLE CHOICE

1. Heat production in the body is primarily a function of:
   a. Metabolism
   b. The skin
   c. The gastrointestinal tract
   d. The kidneys
2. The transfer of heat from a warmer to a cooler environment *not* in direct contact with the body is called:
   a. Evaporation
   b. Conduction
   c. Convection
   d. Radiation
3. The transfer of heat to objects in direct contact with the body is called:
   a. Evaporation
   b. Conduction
   c. Convection
   d. Radiation
4. The transfer of heat to circulating air currents is called:
   a. Evaporation
   b. Conduction
   c. Convection
   d. Radiation
5. The loss of heat when moisture vaporizes on the body surface is called:
   a. Evaporation
   b. Conduction
   c. Convection
   d. Radiation
6. Under normal conditions, most heat loss occurs by:
   a. Evaporation
   b. Conduction
   c. Convection
   d. Radiation
7. Loss of heat by respiration is:
   a. Large
   b. Moderate
   c. Minimal
   d. Not possible
8. The body's "thermostat" that regulates temperature by influencing heat production, heat distribution, and heat loss is located in the:
   a. Cerebellum
   b. Brainstem
   c. Hypothalamus
   d. Pituitary

9. Heat distribution and heat loss are primary responsibilities of the:
   a. Cardiovascular system
   b. Respiratory system
   c. Digestive system
   d. Urinary system
10. When heat loss is needed, the body responds by initiating:
    a. Vasoconstriction
    b. Vasodilation
    c. Shivering
    d. Piloerection
11. High humidity in the environment will decrease the rate of:
    a. Convection
    b. Conduction
    c. Respiration
    d. Evaporation
12. Excessive losses of salt during exercise can cause heat:
    a. Exhaustion
    b. Cramps
    c. Prostration
    d. Stroke
13. Which of the following drinks will help ensure a balanced intake of water and electrolytes?
    a. Sugar water
    b. Gatorade
    c. Orange juice
    d. Seltzer
14. Which of the following age groups is most susceptible to heat emergencies?
    a. Teenagers
    b. Elderly persons
    c. Middle-aged persons
    d. None of the above
15. Alcohol can cause a gain in heat when the environmental temperature is above the body temperature because of:
    a. Vasoconstriction
    b. Vasodilation
    c. Increased pulse
    d. High blood pressure
16. Muscle cramping in heavily used muscles either during or immediately after exertion best describes:
    a. Heat exhaustion
    b. Heat stroke
    c. Heat prostration
    d. Heat cramps

17. The heat disorder that results from widespread vasodilation and fluid loss from sweating is called:
    a. Heat exhaustion
    b. Heat stroke
    c. Heat prostration
    d. Heat cramps
18. On a hot, dry, and windless day (99° F/37° C), the body relies primarily on which of the following mechanisms to lose heat?
    a. Convection
    b. Evaporation
    c. Radiation
    d. Respiration
19. A core body temperature of less than 35° C (95° F) best defines:
    a. Frostbite
    b. Hyperthermia
    c. Hypothermia
    d. Frostnip
20. A normal body response to cold emergencies involves:
    a. Increased metabolism and vasoconstriction
    b. Increased metabolism and vasodilation
    c. Slowed metabolism and vasoconstriction
    d. Slowed metabolism and vasodilation
21. Acute immersion hypothermia is a severe form of cold injury because:
    a. Water is a very good conductor of heat.
    b. Water vapors freeze the nasal mucosa.
    c. Inhalation of water causes bronchoconstriction.
    d. Cold water causes vasodilation and shock.
22. A drug-intoxicated sick person lying on the floor of an apartment (70° F/21° C) for 2 days and becoming hypothermic provides an example of:
    a. Subacute hypothermia
    b. Acute hypothermia
    c. Chronic hypothermia
    d. Frostnip
23. Which of the following statements regarding active external rewarming (placing patient in tub with 105° F/41° C water) is most correct?
    a. It is essential for all patients to avoid brain damage.
    b. It should only be used for severe hypothermia.
    c. It should only be used when transport is significantly delayed.
    d. It should never be used.
24. Which of the following statements regarding stimulation of hypothermic patients is most correct?
    a. They should receive vigorous tactile stimulation so that they do not lapse into a coma.
    b. They should be handled very gently to avoid abnormal heart rhythms.
    c. They should receive strong verbal stimulation to increase circulation to the brain.
    d. They should receive only vigorous stimulation when they are in a coma.

25. For patients with severe hypothermia, hyperventilation should be:
    a. Avoided.
    b. Performed at 24 breaths/min.
    c. Performed at 32 breaths/min.
    d. Performed at 40 breaths/min.
26. Which of the following active rewarming techniques is recommended for field use?
    a. Gastric lavage with warm fluids through nasogastric tube
    b. Warm intravenous fluids and peritoneal lavage
    c. Warmed humidified oxygen and warm packs at arterial points (e.g., armpits)
    d. Use of battery-operated electric blankets
27. Cardiopulmonary resuscitation should be started on hypothermic patients when:
    a. The pulse drops below 50 beats/min.
    b. The pulse drops below 40 beats/min.
    c. The pulse drops below 30 beats/min.
    d. Pulselessness is absolutely certain.
28. A major complication of active external rewarming is:
    a. Burns to the skin.
    b. Respiratory arrest caused by brainstem stimulation.
    c. Rewarming shock caused by vasodilation of peripheral vessels.
    d. Damage to the respiratory mucosa.
29. Which of the following areas of the body is most subject to localized cold injury?
    a. Nose
    b. Genitalia
    c. Legs
    d. Arms
30. Ironically, which of the following mechanisms that protect against hypothermia is the major contributor to localized cold injury?
    a. Increased heart rate
    b. Peripheral vasoconstriction
    c. Shivering
    d. Peripheral vasodilation
31. A completely reversible cold injury characterized by blanching of the skin and loss of sensation in the affected area is called:
    a. Frostbite
    b. Deep
    c. Frostnip
    d. Superficial frostbite
32. A localized cold injury characterized by white, waxy skin that is firm to the touch but with soft, resilient tissue beneath is called:
    a. Deep frostbite
    b. Focal hypothermia
    c. Frostnip
    d. Superficial frostbite

33. The most severe form of localized cold injury that appears white and feels deeply frozen and resists depression to the touch is called:
    a. Deep frostbite
    b. Focal hypothermia
    c. Frostnip
    d. Superficial frostbite

34. Active rewarming of a frostbitten extremity is *not* recommended in the field because:
    a. Of the time needed to effectively rewarm the part.
    b. Arrhythmias may develop.
    c. It can lead to rewarming shock.
    d. It is performed with electrical equipment.

35. If a frostbitten foot should thaw before arrival at the hospital, you should:
    a. Break blisters to relieve pressure.
    b. Cover with sterile dressings.
    c. Encourage the person to walk to improve circulation.
    d. Do nothing to the affected part.

36. In the treatment of poisonous snake bites, attempts to suck out the venom:
    a. Are required in every case.
    b. Remove 90% of the venom.
    c. Are highly controversial.
    d. Should be done after swelling occurs.

37. Which of the following is a useful technique to minimize distribution of the poison of a coral snake bite?
    a. Immobilizing the affected part with an elastic bandage.
    b. Applying an arterial tourniquet.
    c. Using 6 ounces of alcohol.
    d. Placing the part on ice.

MATCHING

Questions 38-41. Match the predisposing factors of heat-related emergencies in column A with the explanations in column B.

Column A	Column B
38. _____ Heart disease	a. Compromised cardiovascular response
39. _____ Obesity	b. Increased insulation results in less heat loss
40. _____ Parkinson disease	c. Inability to care for themselves
41. _____ Mental retardation	d. Muscle tremors produce heat

Questions 42-44. Match the heat-related condition in column A to the signs and symptoms in column B.

Column A	Column B
42. _____ Heat exhaustion	a. Very high temperature, dry skin, altered mental state
43. _____ Heat cramps	b. Muscular cramps after exercise
44. _____ Heat stroke	c. Weakness, cool sweaty skin, rapid pulse, elevated core temperature

Questions 45-51. Categorize the items in column A as either mild, moderate, or severe signs or symptoms of hypothermia in column B.

Column A	Column B
45. _____ Significant hypotension	a. Mild (35°-33° C/ 95°-92° F)
46. _____ Unresponsive to pain	b. Moderate (32°-27° C/ 90°-81° F)
47. _____ Difficulty with speech	c. Severe (26°-22° C/ 79°-72° F)
48. _____ Muscular rigidity	
49. _____ Slowing of pulse and respirations	
50. _____ Ventricular fibrillation	
51. _____ Shivering	

Questions 52-56. Match the distinguishing features in column A with the type of snake in column B.

Column A	Column B
52. _____ Elliptical eyes	a. Nonpoisonous
53. _____ Round eyes	b. Pit viper
54. _____ Pit between eyes and nostrils	
55. _____ Fangs	
56. _____ Triangular head	

Questions 57-60. Match the insect or spider in column A with the identifying characteristics in column B.

Column A	Column B
57. _____ Brown recluse spider	a. Encountered in loose mounds of dirt, and each sting can give rise to a small, circumscribed, elevated lesion.
58. _____ Black widow spider	b. Causes a painful red spot, sometimes with a central blister.
59. _____ Fire ants	c. Severe cases cause problems with vision, swallowing, and slurred speech.
60. _____ Scorpion/ tarantula	d. Causes abdominal pain and lower extremity weakness.

Chapter **16 Environmental Emergencies**

SHORT ANSWER

List the five key questions to ask the patient, or signs that the EMT would look for, in a patient with an environmental emergency.

61. _____

62. _____

63. _____

64. _____

65. _____

TRUE/FALSE

66. _____ A patient with a heat-related emergency is found with moist skin at the time of collapse. Because of this physical finding, it is impossible for the patient to be having heat stroke.

67. _____ The highest priority in treating a patient with heat stroke is rapid transport to the hospital.

68. _____ Some drowning victims die several hours after being removed from the water.

69. _____ Abdominal thrusts should *not* be routinely used in an attempt to clear the lungs of water in a submersion episode.

70. _____ Some patients who drown experience an initial hypoxia caused by laryngeal spasm.

71. _____ The mammalian diving reflex increases metabolism and thus the patient's chance for survival.

CASE SCENARIOS

Questions 72 to 76 refer to the following scenario.
You are on an ice-fishing trip with two friends when you find a hiker who was lost in the woods. He has been walking in deep snowdrifts for the past 3 hours. You bring the hiker into your cabin and examine his feet, which appear white and deeply frozen. It is not possible to evacuate the patient to a hospital for at least 8 more hours.

72. You should:
    a. Keep the extremities frozen until the patient can be transported to the hospital.
    b. Give the patient alcoholic beverages to hasten rewarming.
    c. Begin rewarming of the extremities because of the long transport time.
    d. Rub the extremities vigorously in the snow.

73. Rewarming of a localized cold injury should be performed at a water temperature of:
    a. 100° F/38° C
    b. 102° F/39° C
    c. 105° F/41° C
    d. 110° F/43° C

74. During the active rewarming process, water should:
    a. Remain perfectly still in the container to avoid irritation to the affected part.
    b. Be continuously circulated to maintain an even temperature.
    c. Be allowed to cool to body temperature during the rewarming process.
    d. Be continuously heated slowly up to the patient's tolerance (not to exceed 120° F/49° C).

75. After the rewarming of a deeply frostbitten extremity, pain is:
    a. Common
    b. Very rare
    c. Occasional
    d. Highly unlikely

76. Prolonged exposure (10-12 hours) to above-freezing temperatures and dampness (generally below 10° C/50° F) resulting in cold injury to wet extremities is called:
    a. Deep frostbite
    b. Immersion foot
    c. Frost foot
    d. Cold foot

Question 77 refers to the following scenario.
You respond to a scene and find a 35-year-old man who is unconscious and unresponsive lying on the sidewalk. His temperature is 20° F (−7° C), and you suspect the patient may be experiencing hypothermia.

77. Before beginning cardiac compressions, you should assess for a pulse for:
    a. 5 to 10 seconds
    b. 10 to 20 seconds
    c. 20 to 30 seconds
    d. 30 to 45 seconds

Questions 78 and 79 refer to the following scenario.
A 78-year-old man is found on a park bench on a hot, humid summer day. He is unresponsive to painful stimulus. The physical examination reveals hot, flushed, dry skin and a strong, bounding pulse. His vital signs are respirations 28 beats/min and shallow, pulse 120 beats/min and regular, and blood pressure 190/110 mm Hg.

78. This patient probably has:
    a. A severe infection
    b. Heat stroke
    c. Heat exhaustion
    d. Heat cramps

79. The initial treatment for this patient consists of:
    a. Rapid cooling with alcohol soaks
    b. Rapid cooling with water and convection
    c. Gradual cooling in shade and with saltwater drinks
    d. Rapid transport only

Questions 80 and 81 refer to the following scenario.
You respond to a marathon race and find a 23-year-old man who collapsed during mile 21 of the race on a hot (98° F/37° C) and dry day. Physical examination reveals the patient is lethargic and has pale sweaty skin that is cool to the touch, weakness, dizziness, and a headache. His vital signs are pulse 90 beats/min and regular, respirations 20 breaths/min and shallow, and blood pressure 120/80 mm Hg. However, the blood pressure drops to 90/70 mm Hg when the patient sits up.

80. This patient probably has:
   a. Cardiac syncope
   b. Heat stroke
   c. Heat exhaustion
   d. Heat cramps

81. The initial treatment for this patient consists of:
   a. Rapid cooling with alcohol soaks
   b. Rapid cooling with water and convection
   c. Gradual cooling in the shade and replacement of fluids
   d. Rapid transport only

Questions 82 to 84 refer to the following scenario.
You respond to a schoolyard on a hot, humid day and find a 16-year-old girl complaining of severe leg cramps and sweating profusely. Otherwise, her physical examination and vital signs are normal. The coach tells you that she was running just before the episode.

82. This patient is probably having:
   a. Cardiac syncope
   b. Simple muscle cramps
   c. Heat exhaustion
   d. Heat cramps

83. The primary reason for the cramping is:
   a. Excessive loss of body salt
   b. Widespread vasodilation
   c. Muscle injury
   d. Muscle weakness

84. The initial treatment for this patient consists of:
   a. Rapid cooling with alcohol soaks
   b. Rapid cooling with water and convection
   c. Gradual cooling in shade and fluids
   d. Rapid transport only

Questions 85 and 86 refer to the following scenario.
You respond to an apartment and find a 78-year-old man who fell approximately 2 days ago and was found by his son 30 minutes before your arrival. The room is about 65° F (18° C). Physical examination reveals the patient is responsive to painful but not verbal stimuli; his skin is cool and dry to the touch; and he is shivering slightly. His vital signs are pulse 80 beats/min and irregular, respirations 10 breaths/min and shallow, and blood pressure 90/60 mm Hg.

85. The primary problem with this patient is:
   a. Cardiogenic shock
   b. Shock because of pain in the leg
   c. Cardiac arrhythmia
   d. Moderate hypothermia

86. The initial treatment for this patient consists of:
   a. Warming with blankets
   b. Hot drinks en route to the hospital
   c. Rapid warming with electric blankets
   d. Rapid transport only

Questions 87 to 89 refer to the following scenario.
You respond to a call for a swimming pool injury. At the scene, you find a 7-year-old boy floating supine and slightly submerged in an indoor pool. The patient is unconscious and appears to be cyanotic from the shoulders up. His grandmother (who cannot swim) states that he dove into a shallow part of the pool and did not come up for 2 to 3 minutes.

87. Which of the following treatment considerations should you follow during this boy's removal from the water?
   a. Quick abdominal thrusts as soon as possible
   b. Spinal immobilization precautions
   c. Beginning compressions in the water
   d. Suctioning before ventilation

88. After his removal from the water, what manual airway maneuver would you use to evaluate this boy's breathing?
   a. Head-tilt/chin-lift
   b. Chin pull maneuver
   c. Head-tilt/neck-lift
   d. Jaw thrust without head tilt

89. On removal from the water, you note that the boy's vital signs are pulse 80 beats/min, blood pressure 80/60 mm Hg, and respirations 2 breaths/min. The patient is unresponsive and cyanotic. Your next treatment should be to:
   a. Provide positive-pressure ventilation at a rate of 12 times per minute
   b. Provide positive-pressure ventilation at a rate of 20 times per minute
   c. Place the patient on a nonrebreather oxygen mask
   d. Provide humidified oxygen with a nasal cannula

Questions 90 and 91 refer to the following scenario.
While on standby at an EMS picnic, you are called for a snakebite case. A 24-year-old man was bitten in the ankle by a snake, and his friend killed the snake just before your arrival. You examine the snake and note elliptical eyes, a pit between the eyes and nose, and a triangular head.

90. You conclude that the snake is:
   a. Poisonous
   b. Not poisonous
   c. Poisonous only if it is brightly colored
   d. Poisonous only if it has a rattle tail

91. Your response time to a hospital will be approximately 1 hour. Which of the following actions is appropriate *under these conditions*?
   a. Apply ice to the ankle.
   b. Apply an arterial tourniquet.
   c. Apply an elastic bandage and immobilize the limb.
   d. Cut an "X" at the site of the bite and suck out the venom.

99

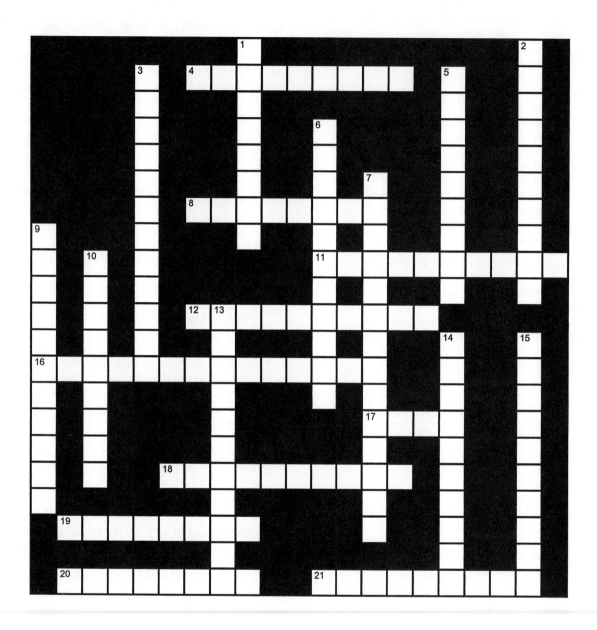

Across

4. Involuntary contraction of small groups of muscles, generating heat
8. Self-administration of drugs, taken in excess or in combination with other agents, to the point of poisoning
11. Life-threatening emergency caused by the victim's inability to sweat
12. Painful muscular contractions of heavily exercised muscles
16. Cardiovascular system's inability to respond to the demands for increased blood flow to the skin while still maintaining flow to the muscles and other organs
17. Organ whose primary role is heat regulation
18. The _____ _____ spider has a red hourglass shape on the abdomen.
19. Reversible cold injury secondary to intense vaso-constriction to cold exposure
20. Suffocation in water or other liquid resulting in death within 24 hours
21. Transfer of heat from a warmer environment to a cooler environment that is not in direct contact with the body

Down

1. Venomous snake with elliptical pupils
2. Venomous snake with red, yellow, and black bands
3. The _____ _____ spider has a dark-colored band on its back resembling a violin.
5. Deep _____ is characterized by freezing extending throughout the dermis and deeper structures, possibly to bone.
6. Core body temperature lower than 35° C/95° F
7. Describes the effects of extremity and shell rewarming before the core temperature can be raised
9. Portion of the brain that sets the body's thermostat and regulates temperature
10. _____ diving reflex
13. Loss of heat that occurs when moisture vaporizes on the body's surface
14. _____ _____ is caused by prolonged exposure to above-freezing temperatures and dampness.
15. Transfer of heat to objects in direct contact with the body.

Chapter **16 Environmental Emergencies**

17 Behavioral Emergencies

MULTIPLE CHOICE

1. Which of the following age groups are most likely to commit suicide?
   a. Small children
   b. Persons in their 20s
   c. Middle-aged women
   d. Elderly men

2. You have a confused and agitated patient in your ambulance who thinks that he is in church and that you are his son. Your best approach would be to:
   a. Quietly go along with what he is saying so that he will not become more agitated.
   b. Tell him that you are an EMT, and that he is in an ambulance on the way to a hospital.
   c. Let him think you are his son, but tell him where he is.
   d. Restrain the patient, and do not try to talk to him.

3. An emotional response to a sudden illness, death in the family, or other difficult personal experience, accompanied by anxiety, fear, paranoia, anger, hysteria, denial, or withdrawal, is called a:
   a. Situational reaction
   b. Nervous breakdown
   c. Hysterical reaction
   d. Temporary breach

4. Nervousness, tension, pacing, hand wringing, and trembling are all symptoms of:
   a. Anxiety
   b. Paranoia
   c. Hysteria
   d. Suicidal tendencies

5. A patient who is afraid that you are trying to kill him with poison gas when you place an oxygen mask over his face may be experiencing:
   a. Anxiety
   b. Confusion
   c. Paranoia
   d. Hysteria

6. A patient who is having a heart attack and does *not* want to go in the ambulance because he "just has a little chest pain" most likely is experiencing:
   a. Denial
   b. Hysteria
   c. Anxiety
   d. Confusion

7. A patient who has difficulty sleeping, loss of appetite, loss of sex drive, inability to feel pleasure, and feelings of hopelessness most likely is experiencing:
   a. Denial
   b. Depression
   c. Hysteria
   d. Psychosis

8. A person who is about to commit suicide:
   a. Always exhibits signs of depression.
   b. Never calls for help.
   c. May appear very content and even happy.
   d. Is never a danger to others.

9. Distorted perceptions of reality, with hallucinations and inappropriate responses to the environment, best describe a:
   a. Phobia
   b. Situational reaction
   c. Psychosis
   d. Hysterical reaction

10. The first priority when faced with an emotionally disturbed patient is to:
    a. Restrain the patient immediately.
    b. Consider possible medical causes.
    c. Give sedation and then restrain the patient.
    d. Obtain permission from the family to restrain the patient.

11. The first priority with a potentially dangerous patient is:
    a. Self-protection
    b. The patient's protection
    c. The legal implications
    d. Restraining the patient

12. A suicidal patient who is explaining her reasons for wanting to commit suicide should be managed by:
    a. Comparing her problems to those of others, thus minimizing their severity.
    b. Acknowledging her perspective and offering her help at the hospital.
    c. Being firm and taking a "parental role" in your relationship with her.
    d. Waiting for an opportunity, then quickly restraining her with police assistance.

13. In general, the best posture to assume when dealing with a violent patient is:
    a. Firm and authoritative
    b. Aggressive and self-assured
    c. Calm and reassuring
    d. Lighthearted and carefree

14. Responses such as guilt, grief, anger, hysteria, denial, withdrawal, and physical reactions are common reactions to:
    a. Phobias
    b. Pain
    c. Organic illness
    d. Death
15. A situation in which a patient exhibits behavior that is unacceptable or intolerable to the patient, family, or community best describes a(n):
    a. Anxiety reaction
    b. Psychobehavioral disorder
    c. Psychosis
    d. Schizophrenic reaction
16. You encounter a 48-year-old patient exhibiting violent behavior who attempted to cut his wrists and now refuses to go to the hospital. After multiple attempts to convince him with a calm reassuring approach, you should:
    a. Work with police to restrain and remove the patient.
    b. Allow the patient to refuse care because he is an adult.
    c. Leave him alone with family members to convince him.
    d. Use a contrived story to convince him to go.

SHORT ANSWER

Questions 17-23. List the seven key questions to ask the patient with a behavioral emergency.

17. _____
    _____
18. _____
    _____
19. _____
    _____
20. _____
    _____
21. _____
    _____
22. _____
    _____
23. _____
    _____

Questions 24-31. List the eight common medical and environmental causes of behavioral alteration.

24. _____
25. _____
26. _____
27. _____
28. _____
29. _____
30. _____
31. _____

TRUE/FALSE

32. _____ Suicide is the eleventh leading cause of death in the United States.
33. _____ Paranoia is the most common mental disorder in elderly patients.
34. _____ A person about to commit suicide always shows signs of depression.
35. _____ The most important aspect of the initial assessment of the patient with a suspected behavioral emergency is to look for the possibility of an underlying medical cause.
36. _____ Visual, tactile (touch), or olfactory (smell) hallucinations almost always have an organic cause.

CASE SCENARIOS

Questions 37 and 38 refer to the following scenario.
You have a female patient who appears to have been badly beaten and possibly raped. She refuses to answer questions about where she is hurt or what happened to her. She simply stares into space and refuses to look at you.

37. This patient's common reaction to a traumatic situation is known as:
    a. Denial
    b. Withdrawal
    c. Confusion
    d. Hysteria
38. Your first action in caring for this patient should be to:
    a. Examine her to see if she was raped.
    b. Identify yourself in a gentle and reassuring manner.
    c. Focus on injuries, not emotional issues.
    d. Have her describe the incident so she can experience an emotional catharsis.

Questions 39 and 40 refer to the following scenario.
You respond to a residence and find a patient who is combative and angry. His family states that he suddenly exhibited aggressive and dangerous behavior, but that he never behaves in this manner. The past medical history indicates no psychiatric disorders, but the patient has a history of heart disease, diabetes, and chronic obstructive lung disease.

39. This patient's condition is most likely related to:
    a. Psychosis
    b. Depression

c. Hypoglycemia
d. A drug reaction

40. Your action in caring for this patient should include:
    a. Administering glucose.
    b. Administering epinephrine.
    c. Restraining the patient with police and family.
    d. Inducing vomiting.

Questions 41 and 42 refer to the following scenario.
You are dispatched to a call for a patient with terminal cancer. At the scene, you encounter a 34-year-old patient dying from leukemia. The patient is conscious and aware of his condition. He responds angrily to almost every request or comment made to him.

41. This patient's reaction:
    a. Is very common with dying patients.
    b. Suggests insensitivity on your part.
    c. Must be dealt with firmly.
    d. Should be actively converted by cheerfulness.

42. The most effective method for dealing with this patient is:
    a. Empathetic listening
    b. Firm interaction and directions
    c. A detached clinical approach
    d. Distraction from his problems

Questions 43 to 45 refer to the following scenario.
You respond to the scene of an apartment house fire and encounter a 33-year-old man who is being restrained by the police. He tells you that his wife and two children are still trapped in the building. You continue to stay with this person until the fire is under control.

43. Your patient is tense and cannot stay still. He continues to pace back and forth as he watches the efforts of the fire department to find his family. This patient is exhibiting signs of:
    a. Anxiety
    b. Paranoia
    c. Agitation
    d. Denial

44. Approximately 30 minutes elapse, and the fire chief comes over and tells your patient that the bodies of his wife and two children have been found. Your patient begins to cry uncontrollably and starts beating his fists against a car. This patient is now exhibiting signs of:
    a. Anxiety
    b. Paranoia
    c. Agitation
    d. Denial

45. You continue to comfort your patient and offer to call a friend or relative to be with him. Initially the patient ignores you and then sits on the ground with his head in his hands. You continue to reassure the patient, but he is refusing to talk or interact with you. This patient is now exhibiting signs of:
    a. Anxiety
    b. Paranoia
    c. Agitation
    d. Withdrawal

Chapter **17 Behavioral Emergencies**

18 Abuse and Assault

MULTIPLE CHOICE

1. The first consideration when arriving at the scene of suspected domestic violence is:
   a. Ensuring scene safety.
   b. Providing airway management.
   c. Determining the number of patients.
   d. Obtaining a general impression of the patient.
2. You respond at a middle school and are caring for a 13-year-old boy who reportedly fell from a swing when you notice purplish bruises on his thighs and welts on his back. The patient tells you that he fell a few days ago and sustained these injuries. You should:
   a. Refuse to transport the patient until his parents arrive at the scene.
   b. Treat the patient but not document suspicion of abuse because the patient has denied that abuse occurred.
   c. Not call child protective services or report the incident because you would be liable if you reported suspected abuse and no abuse actually occurred.
   d. Transport the patient to the hospital, inform the staff of your suspicions of abuse, and report the suspected abuse to the appropriate agency.

SHORT ANSWER

Questions 3-5. List the three phases of the cycle of violence in order of occurrence.

3. _____

4. _____

5. _____

Questions 6-15. List 10 signs of physical abuse.

6. _____

7. _____

8. _____

9. _____

10. _____

11. _____

12. _____

13. _____

14. _____

15. _____

Questions 16 and 17. List two key clues (not physical signs) that should raise the index of suspicion of abuse.

16. _____

17. _____

Questions 18-22. List five nonphysical signs or symptoms of psychological or emotional abuse.

18. _____

19. _____

20. _____

21. _____

22. _____

Questions 23-30. List eight indicators of neglect that may be seen when treating and evaluating an elderly patient.

23. _____

24. _____

25. _____

26. _____

27. _____

28. _____

29. _____

30. _____

TRUE/FALSE

31. _____ Abused women are more likely to seek prenatal care.

32. _____ Women whose pregnancies were unwanted are less likely to experience physical violence.

33. _____ The infliction of psychological or emotional abuse is termed assault.

34. _____ Children whose mothers were victims of wife battery are twice as likely to be abused themselves as those children whose mothers were not victims of abuse.

35. _____ The majority of elder abuse victims are men.

36. _____ Performing a physical assessment is unlikely to determine any signs of abuse.

CASE SCENARIO

Questions 37 and 38 refer to the following scenario.
You respond to an apartment complex and encounter a 32-year-old woman at a friend's apartment who states that she was raped at her apartment in another building. Your general impression of the patient reveals a small contusion on her forehead. The patient does not have any other physical complaints. Her blood pressure is 122/76 mm Hg, heart rate 76 beats/min (regular and strong), and respiratory rate 12 breaths/min and normal. Skin color, temperature, and condition are normal, and her pupils are equal and react to light.

37. The patient tells you that before transport to the hospital, she wants to go back to her apartment to "clean up." You inform her that:
    a. She can change her clothes, but she should not shower.
    b. She should not wash, change her clothes, or urinate until she is examined at the hospital.
    c. It is appropriate for her to shower and change, and her family can transport her to the hospital when she is ready.
    d. She should douche immediately to minimize the possibility of becoming pregnant.

38. During treatment of this patient you should:
    a. Cut away her clothing as you examine her.
    b. Remove her clothing as you examine her.
    c. Perform only a physical assessment that focuses on assessing and treating life-threatening problems.
    d. Ask the patient to describe her attacker and all aspects of her assault.

19 Obstetrics and Gynecology

MULTIPLE CHOICE

1. A major function of the fallopian tubes is:
   a. Carrying eggs from the ovary to the uterus
   b. The site of implantation of a normal pregnancy
   c. The connecting point between the cervix and the vagina
   d. The site of egg production
2. The part of the body where eggs are stored and become mature and where female hormones are produced is the:
   a. Fallopian tube
   b. Uterus
   c. Ovary
   d. Cervix
3. The section of the uterus that dilates during labor is the:
   a. Body
   b. Cervix
   c. Fundus
   d. Myometrium
4. The organ through which nutrients and waste products are exchanged between the fetus and the mother is the:
   a. Uterus
   b. Placenta
   c. Liver
   d. Cervix
5. The umbilical cord contains:
   a. One vein and one artery
   b. One vein and two arteries
   c. Two veins and one artery
   d. Two veins and two arteries
6. The first stage of labor:
   a. Begins with full dilation of the cervix and ends when the baby is born.
   b. Lasts from the onset of contractions until the cervix is completely dilated.
   c. Ends at the onset of transition.
   d. Should never last more than 1 hour.
7. During the second stage of labor:
   a. The mother often has an urge to move her bowels.
   b. Postpartum hemorrhage may occur.
   c. You can expect to deliver the placenta.
   d. Labor contractions stop.
8. Your first action after the baby's head is born is to:
   a. Clamp the cord.
   b. Suction the baby's mouth and nose with a bulb syringe.
   c. Dry the baby thoroughly.
   d. Deliver the placenta.

9. During a normal vertex delivery, as soon as the baby's head is born, your second action is to:
   a. Immediately tell the mother to push before the cervix closes.
   b. Ask the mother to pant while you check to see if there is a cord wrapped around the baby's neck.
   c. Examine the mouth to see if the baby has a cleft lip.
   d. Tell the mother to push.
10. If a baby's head is born and you find that the umbilical cord is wrapped tightly around the baby's neck, you should:
    a. Give the mother oxygen and transport rapidly.
    b. Stretch the cord over the baby's head to unwind it.
    c. Clamp the cord close together in two places and cut between the clamps.
    d. Try to push the head back inside slightly to ease tension around the baby's neck.
11. In a vertex delivery with meconium-stained fluid, the infant's mouth:
    a. Should be suctioned only after the nose is suctioned.
    b. Should be suctioned before stimulating the baby to breathe.
    c. Should be suctioned only after you check the heart rate.
    d. Should not be suctioned because you will contaminate the mouth with bacteria.
12. When you find the baby's leg projecting from the vagina in a laboring patient, you should:
    a. Grasp the leg firmly and pull until you can reach the other leg.
    b. Transport rapidly while giving oxygen to the mother.
    c. Try to push the leg back inside the vagina.
    d. Press on the mother's fundus and ask her to push.
13. After a baby is born and the cord is cut, you notice a sudden gush of blood from the mother's vagina and lengthening of the umbilical cord. This would indicate:
    a. Laceration of the vagina
    b. The onset of a postpartum hemorrhage
    c. The placenta is about to deliver
    d. Uterine rupture
14. Allowing the mother to nurse a healthy, full-term newborn after birth:
    a. Should never be done in the ambulance.
    b. Can help to contract the uterus.
    c. Can relieve cyanosis in a newborn.
    d. Supplies the newborn with needed calories.

109

15. If the placenta does *not* spontaneously deliver by the time the baby is wrapped and the mother has been cleaned, you should:
    a. Ask the mother to push while you pull on the cord.
    b. Proceed to the hospital.
    c. Ask the mother to stand; gravity may deliver the placenta.
    d. Perform the knee-chest maneuver.

16. When resuscitating a newborn, the heart rate is counted:
    a. For a full minute
    b. For 6 seconds
    c. Only after the Apgar score is done
    d. For 30 seconds

17. Positive-pressure ventilation for a newborn should be done at a rate of:
    a. 20 to 30 breaths/min
    b. 40 to 60 breaths/min
    c. 80 to 100 breaths/min
    d. 120 to 140 breaths/min

18. The concentration of oxygen for positive-pressure ventilation of a newborn should be:
    a. 90% to 100%
    b. 50% to 60%
    c. 24% to 36%
    d. Never give oxygen to a newborn.

19. Chest compressions in the newborn should be:
    a. One-third the anterior-posterior depth of chest at 100 compressions/min
    b. One-third the anterior-posterior depth of chest at 120 compressions/min
    c. Half the anterior-posterior depth of chest at 100 compressions/min
    d. Half the anterior-posterior depth of chest at 120 compressions/min

20. A newborn is breathing at birth, so you check the heart rate, 80 beats/min. Your next action would be to:
    a. Evaluate the baby's color.
    b. Begin positive-pressure ventilation with 100% oxygen.
    c. Begin cardiac compressions.
    d. Give 100% free-flow oxygen.

21. When resuscitating a newborn, cardiac compressions should be discontinued once the baby's heart rate is more than:
    a. 60 beats/min
    b. 80 beats/min
    c. 90 beats/min
    d. 100 beats/min

22. An infant born with a cleft palate:
    a. Will probably also be brain-damaged.
    b. Should not be allowed to nurse.
    c. Should not be shown to the mother.
    d. All of the above.

23. Allowing the newborn to become chilled can:
    a. Help establish respirations if the baby does not cry.
    b. Cause hypoglycemia and acidosis.
    c. Stimulate a more rapid heart rate as the baby tries to stay warm.
    d. Help to keep the baby awake so he or she can nurse.

24. In general, the position for transport of a pregnant patient in her third trimester is:
    a. Supine
    b. Prone
    c. On her left side
    d. On her right side

25. The reason for transporting a pregnant woman in this position (see question 24) is:
    a. You always want to have the mother facing you in the ambulance.
    b. Most babies are facing the mother's right side late in pregnancy, and pressure on the back of the baby's head can dangerously lower the heart rate.
    c. To prevent damage to the liver.
    d. The vena cava is right of the midline, and you do not want to compress it between the spinal column and the weight of the baby.

26. During normal pregnancy the blood pressure:
    a. Should not change.
    b. Becomes slightly higher than before pregnancy.
    c. Becomes much higher than before pregnancy.
    d. Becomes lower than before pregnancy.

27. A baby born to a diabetic mother:
    a. Is often large, and delivery can be complicated.
    b. Is prone to hyperglycemia after delivery.
    c. Is not usually affected by the mother's disease.
    d. Will probably be born with diabetes.

28. The points assigned for each APGAR category range from:
    a. 0 to 2
    b. 1 to 3
    c. 1 to 5
    d. 1 to 6

29. Maternal hypertension is defined as blood pressure of:
    a. Systolic greater than 180 or diastolic greater than 100 mm Hg
    b. Systolic greater than 160 or diastolic greater than 100 mm Hg
    c. Systolic greater than 150 or diastolic greater than 90 mm Hg
    d. Systolic greater than 140 or diastolic greater than 90 mm Hg

30. Preeclampsia becomes eclampsia when:
    a. Hypertension and edema are both present.
    b. The blood pressure exceeds 180/100 mm Hg.
    c. A seizure occurs.
    d. All of the above.

31. If you examine a laboring patient and find the umbilical cord bulging out of the vagina, you should:
    a. Clamp and cut the cord so that the baby can be delivered.
    b. Try to elevate the presenting part with a gloved hand so it does not compress the cord.
    c. Gently place the cord back inside the vagina.
    d. Place a moist pressure dressing over the vagina.
32. Prolapsed cord is often associated with:
    a. Placenta previa
    b. Abruptio placentae
    c. Abnormal presentation, such as breech or shoulder
    d. Preeclampsia
33. You arrive at a call to find a patient who states she is approximately 32 weeks' pregnant, but she has *not* seen a physician because she has no money. She awoke in the middle of the night and was very upset to find that she had passed a good deal of bright-red blood from her vagina. She has no abdominal or pelvic tenderness but complains of mild, low back pain. Her skin is pale, warm, and dry to the touch. Her vital signs are blood pressure 100/56 mm Hg, pulse 108 beats/min, and respirations 22 breaths/min. Your first action would be to:
    a. Do a gentle vaginal examination to see if the patient is about to deliver.
    b. Place the patient on her left side and give high-concentration oxygen.
    c. Insert a pressure dressing into the vagina to control the bleeding.
    d. Massage the patient's uterus to control the bleeding.
34. You arrive at a call to find a woman who is 30 weeks' pregnant with her second child. She complains of labor pains but cannot say how far apart they are because the pain is almost constant. Her uterus feels hard, and she is restless and crying from the pain. History reveals that she was in a motor vehicle accident yesterday, was seen in the emergency department, and was treated for sprained wrists (bracing against dashboard). She was a front-seat passenger wearing a lap belt restraint. There is no vaginal bleeding or discharge. Her vital signs are blood pressure 130/80 mm Hg, pulse 114 beats/min, and respirations 24 breaths/min. Your best action for this patient would be to:
    a. Take out an obstetric kit and prepare for a premature delivery.
    b. Place her on her left side, give oxygen, and transport immediately.
    c. Do a vaginal examination to see if the cervix is dilated.
    d. Use the knee-chest maneuver.

35. A patient complains of severe shoulder pain that came on suddenly. Physical examination reveals abdominal tenderness, and she is starting to have some vaginal bleeding. Her skin is pale, cool, and clammy. She missed her last period. This patient's symptoms are most likely caused by:
    a. Placenta previa
    b. Threatened abortion
    c. Ruptured ectopic pregnancy
    d. Breech presentation
36. You arrive at a call to find a patient in labor. She is very uncomfortable, with contractions occurring every 3 minutes and lasting 60 seconds. She is restless and demands to go to the bathroom. Physical examination reveals a slight bulging of the perineum and rectum, but no presenting part is visible. There is a gush of fluid during a contraction, and you note that the fluid is meconium stained. Your best action for this patient would be to:
    a. Explain that the urge to go to the bathroom is probably the baby coming, then have the woman lie on her bed and prepare for a delivery.
    b. Allow her to go to the bathroom so that she will be more cooperative.
    c. Explain that the urge to go to the bathroom is probably the baby coming, then get her to lie on the stretcher in the ambulance and prepare for a delivery en route to the hospital.
    d. Put the mother in the knee-chest position.
37. Proper body substance isolation procedures for a childbirth include:
    a. Gloves only
    b. Gloves and goggles
    c. Gloves, goggles, and mask
    d. Gloves, goggles, and gown
38. An explosive delivery is best prevented by:
    a. Applying gentle pressure to the crown of the baby's head during delivery.
    b. Elevating the mother's hips during delivery.
    c. Performing the knee-chest maneuver.
    d. Applying gentle downward pressure on the shoulders.
39. Premature babies are at very high risk for:
    a. Respiratory problems and hypothermia
    b. Meconium aspiration
    c. Ventricular fibrillation
    d. Cleft palate
40. As a general rule, how long should you wait before transport for the second baby to deliver in a mother who is expecting twins?
    a. 3 minutes
    b. 5 minutes
    c. 10 minutes
    d. 30 minutes

Chapter **19 Obstetrics and Gynecology**

FILL IN THE BLANK

41. The Apgar score is performed at 1 minute after

    birth and is repeated _____ after birth.
42. You should hold the oxygen tubing approximately

    _____ from the infant's nose when
    administering free-flow oxygen.
43. The volume of air in the lungs of a newborn is

    approximately _____.

SHORT ANSWER

Questions 44-50. List the seven questions to ask the patient with an obstetric emergency.

44. _____

    _____
45. _____

    _____
46. _____

    _____
47. _____

    _____
48. _____

    _____
49. _____

    _____
50. _____

    _____

Questions 51 and 52. List two causes of left shoulder pain in a woman with no history of trauma.

51. _____

    _____
52. _____

    _____

Questions 53-56. List four signs of respiratory distress in the newborn.

53. _____

    _____
54. _____

    _____
55. _____

    _____
56. _____

    _____

Questions 57-61. List the five components of the Apgar score.

57. A _____

    _____
58. P _____

    _____
59. G _____

    _____
60. A _____

    _____
61. R _____

    _____

CASE SCENARIOS

Questions 62 to 64 refer to the following scenario.
You arrive at a call and find a 34-year-old woman who has just delivered her third child, a full-term girl. A survey of the newborn reveals a healthy infant with well-established respirations and no signs of distress. The placenta delivers spontaneously, and you are about to transport the patient when the vaginal bleeding becomes very heavy. The mother's blood pressure is 90/50 mm Hg, pulse 118 beats/min, and respirations 22 breaths/min. Her skin is cool, somewhat clammy, and pale.

62. The most common cause of early postpartum hemorrhage is:
    a. Perineal lacerations
    b. Uterine atony
    c. Ruptured uterus
    d. Prolapsed uterus
63. Your first action for this patient would be to:
    a. Apply direct pressure to the perineum.
    b. Palpate and massage the uterus.
    c. Elevate the patient's hips.
    d. Apply an ice pack to the perineum.
64. Postpartum hemorrhage is defined as blood loss of, or greater than:
    a. 100 mL
    b. 500 mL
    c. 800 mL
    d. 1000 mL

Questions 65 and 66 refer to the following scenario.
You arrive at a call to find a 19-year-old woman who has been beaten and raped by a stranger. Her clothes are torn and bloodstained, and she is crying.

65. The best way to proceed in this situation is:
    a. Gently help the woman to change her clothes and wash up, then transport her.
    b. Gently assess for further injuries, treat as necessary, and transport her.
    c. Examine her perineum to assess for injuries.
    d. Encourage her to douche before going to the hospital to prevent infection.

66. The best attitude to take with this patient is to:
    a. Minimize the event so that it does not seem so bad.
    b. Be gentle, understanding, and compassionate.
    c. Talk to her as little as possible.
    d. Be authoritative because she needs to feel someone is in control.

Questions 67 to 70 refer to the following scenario.
You have a patient whose chief complaints are epigastric pain, headache, and dizziness. She is about 30 weeks' pregnant and has marked puffiness in her hands, legs, and face. As you lift the stretcher, she starts to complain of blurred vision. Her vital signs are blood pressure 170/100 mm Hg, pulse 122 beats/min, and respirations 24 breaths/min.

67. This patient probably has:
    a. Diabetes
    b. Heart attack
    c. Preeclampsia
    d. Gastric ulcer

68. Your best action for this patient would be to:
    a. Put on lights and sirens and rush to the hospital.
    b. Place her on her left side, give oxygen, have suction equipment ready, and proceed quietly to the hospital.
    c. Ask her to push so you can deliver the baby.
    d. Give her milk to drink to relieve the gastric acidity.

69. The dizziness, blurred vision, and headache are probably caused by:
    a. Cerebral and retinal edema
    b. Gastric ulcer
    c. Hypoglycemia
    d. Shock

70. There is a good possibility that this patient may soon have a:
    a. Cardiac arrest
    b. Full gastric bleed
    c. Seizure
    d. Hypoglycemic reaction

Questions 71 to 75 refer to the following scenario.
You arrive at an obstetric call to find that a breech delivery is in progress. The patient is a 28-year-old woman who tells you that this is her third pregnancy. The baby has been born up to the neck.

71. Which of the following is almost always present in a breech delivery?
    a. A premature baby
    b. Meconium fluid
    c. An umbilical cord around the neck
    d. Heavy vaginal bleeding

72. The mother is pushing uncontrollably, but the head will not deliver. To assist, you might:
    a. Twist the baby's body around until the head pops out.
    b. Place your fingers on both sides of the baby's nose and flex the baby's chin on the chest.
    c. Clamp and cut the umbilical cord.
    d. Place the mother on her left side and ask her to stop pushing.

73. The baby requires positive-pressure ventilation. The percentage of oxygen given during positive-pressure ventilation is:
    a. 100%
    b. 80%
    c. 50%
    d. 21%

74. After 30 seconds of positive-pressure ventilation, your partner checks the baby's heart rate, 50 beats/min. The EMT should now:
    a. Discontinue positive-pressure ventilation.
    b. Continue positive-pressure ventilation and begin chest compressions.
    c. Stimulate the baby if breathing.
    d. Suction the baby's mouth and nostrils.

75. The baby has been successfully resuscitated. You notice that his right arm hangs limply at his side, with no grasp reflex in the hand. This is probably caused by:
    a. Brain damage
    b. Damage to the brachial nerves
    c. Hypoglycemia
    d. Dislocation of the shoulder

Questions 76 to 80 refer to the following scenario.
You respond to a call at a shopping mall and encounter a 23-year-old woman who informs you that she is 32 weeks' pregnant with her second child. She was walking in the mall when her water broke, and she immediately began to feel contractions. You place the patient in a security area out of public view and begin your evaluation. On visual examination you note that the baby's head is visible in the vagina with each contraction. The patient asks permission to use the bathroom because she has a strong urge to move her bowels.

76. Based on your examination, you should:
    a. Escort the patient to the bathroom.
    b. Begin transport to the hospital and allow the patient to use a bedpan.
    c. Prepare for imminent delivery of the baby.
    d. Place the patient in the knee-chest position on the stretcher and begin rapid transport to the hospital.

77. After your initial steps in treating the baby, your evaluation reveals that the baby is not breathing. Your immediate response is to:
    a. Provide positive-pressure ventilations and CPR compressions.
    b. Provide positive-pressure ventilations without CPR compressions.
    c. Deliver supplemental oxygen with an infant oxygen mask.
    d. Deliver supplemental oxygen with oxygen supply tubing.

78. After 30 seconds of respiratory therapy the infant starts to cry. Your next action is to:
    a. Check the heart rate and give free-flow oxygen.
    b. Provide positive-pressure ventilations.
    c. Start chest compressions.
    d. Suction the infant.

113

79. While you continue to treat the baby, you notice that your partner delivers the placenta. The placenta delivers during the:
   a. First stage of labor
   b. Second stage of labor
   c. Third stage of labor
   d. Fourth stage of labor

80. After the placenta is delivered, the patient continues to bleed heavily from the vagina. You evaluate the patient, and you do not see any external tears in the perineum, but bleeding continues to come from the vagina. You should:
   a. Apply the pneumatic antishock garment and transport.
   b. Massage the uterus.
   c. Allow the baby to nurse, place the patient on her left side, and transport rapidly.
   d. Apply dressings and transport immediately.

CROSSWORD PUZZLE

Puzzle 19-1

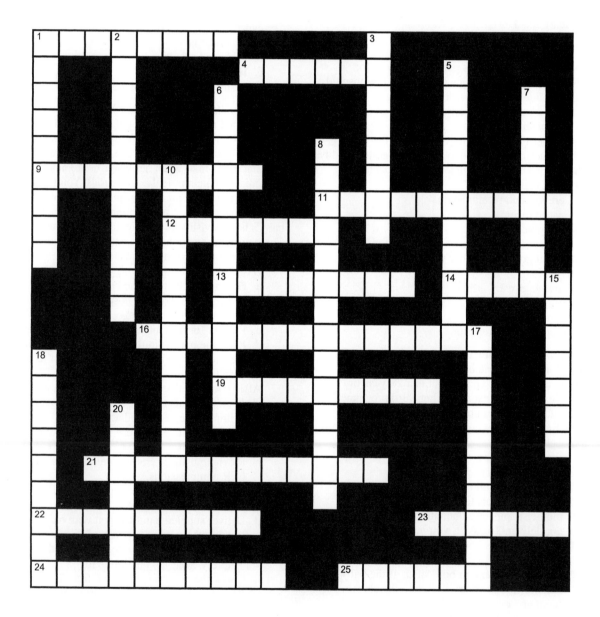

Across

1. Feces found in amniotic fluid alerting to a stressed fetus
4. Home for the developing fetus
9. Condition characterized by high blood pressure and seizures
11. Absence or cessation of menstrual period
12. Pregnancy occurring outside the uterus
13. Appearance of the full diameter of fetal head through birth canal
14. _____ score is a system used to rapidly evaluate a newborn.
16. Trumpet-shaped structures assisting with mature egg movement
19. Uterine _____ is a condition requiring replacement of the uterus into the vagina.
21. Sign of respiratory distress in newborns
22. Vein that carries oxygenated blood to the fetus
23. Lowest segment of the uterus
24. An incision, made by the physician, to facilitate easier delivery
25. Presentation of buttocks first into the pelvis

Down

1. Maneuver used to assist in releasing a wedged anterior shoulder of baby during delivery.
2. Nontraumatic, severe shoulder pain in a woman of childbearing age may be caused by _____
3. Hormone vital to menstruation and pregnancy
5. Loss of pregnancy before 20 weeks' gestation
6. Watery liquid that protects the fetus
7. Afterbirth
8. Growth of placenta over part or all of the cervical opening
10. High blood pressure and edema during pregnancy
15. Uterine _____ may occur after a previous cesarean birth or trauma.
17. Loss of pregnancy after 20 weeks' gestation
18. Infant less than 5½ pounds or 37 weeks' gestation
20. Glands where eggs are produced

Chapter **19** **Obstetrics and Gynecology**

20 Bleeding and Shock

MULTIPLE CHOICE

1. Failure of the circulatory system to adequately perfuse and oxygenate the tissues of the body best defines:
   a. Respiratory failure
   b. Shock
   c. Heart failure
   d. Clinical death
2. The "fight or flight" response is mediated by:
   a. Atropine
   b. Epinephrine (adrenaline)
   c. Histamine
   d. Dopamine
3. Which of the following is an effect of epinephrine (adrenaline) release?
   a. Decreased heart rate
   b. Constriction of the pupils
   c. Increased force of heart contraction
   d. Decreased blood flow to the brain
4. Shock that occurs from a myocardial infarction (heart attack) is called:
   a. Cardiogenic shock
   b. Distributive shock
   c. Obstructive shock
   d. Hypovolemic shock
5. Which of the following is most likely to result in a vasodilatory type of shock?
   a. Anaphylaxis
   b. Hemorrhage
   c. Tension pneumothorax
   d. Heart attack
6. Which of the following conditions may cause hypovolemic shock?
   a. Coronary thrombosis
   b. Anaphylaxis
   c. Myocardial infarction
   d. Diabetes
7. A condition characterized by a low supply of hemoglobin is:
   a. Hypotensive syndrome
   b. Anemia
   c. Ischemia
   d. Hypovolemia
8. Bleeding characterized by pulsatile flow and bright-red blood is:
   a. Capillary
   b. Venous
   c. Systemic
   d. Arterial
9. Which of the following is a characteristic of venous bleeding?
   a. Pulsatile flow
   b. Dark-red color
   c. Occurs in deep wounds
   d. Always requires pressure point to control
10. The first step used to control bleeding is:
    a. Pressure point
    b. Tourniquet
    c. Air splint
    d. Direct pressure
11. Which of the following steps of bleeding control should be done as the *final* method?
    a. Direct pressure
    b. Tourniquet
    c. Pressure point
    d. Elevation
12. The pressure point for the upper extremity is located over the:
    a. Femoral artery
    b. Radial artery
    c. Ulnar artery
    d. Brachial artery
13. The pressure point for the lower extremity is located over the:
    a. Femoral artery
    b. Radial artery
    c. Ulnar artery
    d. Brachial artery
14. The first compensatory response of the body to acute blood loss (less than 15%) is:
    a. Venous constriction
    b. Hypotension
    c. Arterial constriction
    d. None of the above
15. Which of the following signs is the *last* to occur after acute blood loss?
    a. Pale skin
    b. Tachycardia
    c. Delayed capillary refill
    d. Hypotension
16. Which of the following best describes the sequence of the signs of hypovolemic shock?
    a. Altered mental status, rapid pulse, hypotension, delayed capillary refill
    b. Hypotension, rapid pulse, delayed capillary refill, altered mental status
    c. Rapid pulse, delayed capillary refill, hypotension, altered mental status
    d. Rapid pulse, altered mental status, hypotension, delayed capillary refill

117

17. Use of the abdominal section of the pneumatic antishock garment (PASG) is contraindicated in the presence of:
    a. Penetrating chest injury
    b. Suspected ruptured spleen
    c. Contusions on abdominal wall
    d. Kidney injuries
18. The PASG is primarily used in the prehospital treatment of which form of shock?
    a. Cardiogenic shock
    b. Distributive shock
    c. Obstructive shock
    d. Hypovolemic shock
19. When removing the PASG in the hospital, you should:
    a. Remove them quickly starting with the legs.
    b. Remove them quickly starting with the abdominal section.
    c. Remove them slowly while monitoring blood pressure.
    d. Remove them slowly while monitoring garment pressure.
20. Which of the following is a possible effect of the PASG?
    a. Increases peripheral vascular resistance.
    b. Tamponades bleeding in the chest.
    c. Transfuses large amounts of blood to torso.
    d. Shunts blood to the extremities.
21. The upper margin of the abdominal section of the PASG should be placed no higher than the:
    a. Umbilicus
    b. Iliac crest of pelvis
    c. Lower margin of rib cage
    d. Suprapubic region
22. Which of the following is a contraindication to the use of the PASG?
    a. Intraabdominal bleeding
    b. Pelvic injury
    c. Extremity bleeding
    d. Chest injury
23. If a patient had severe bleeding in the face and mouth, your greatest immediate concern would be:
    a. Control of the airway
    b. Severe blood loss
    c. Brain injury
    d. Injury to the eyes
24. The appropriate body substance isolation procedures for a patient with a spurting wound would be:
    a. Gloves only
    b. Gloves and goggles
    c. Gloves, goggles, and mask
    d. Gloves, goggles, mask, and gown

FILL IN THE BLANK

25. The amount of blood pumped out of the heart with each beat is called the _____ _____.

26. The amount of blood pumped by the heart each minute is called the _____ _____.

27. Stroke volume multiplied by _____ _____ equals cardiac output.

28. The force exerted by the blood volume on the walls of the vessels is called the _____ _____.

TRUE/FALSE

29. _____ The most effective treatment for cardiogenic shock is the PASG.
30. _____ Infants and children may maintain their blood pressure until their blood volume is more than half depleted.
31. _____ When the systolic blood pressure is identified as 120, the number 120 refers to psi (pounds per square inch).
32. _____ The release of epinephrine causes the pupils to constrict.
33. _____ A patient with a closed fracture of the femur may lose approximately 1 L of blood at the injury site.
34. _____ A partially severed artery is most likely to clot because of the high volume of blood flowing through it.
35. _____ When controlling bleeding from the nose, the patient should be positioned sitting and leaning forward if there is no suspected neck or back injury.

CASE SCENARIOS

Questions 36 to 38 refer to the following scenario.
You respond to a call and find a 26-year-old man who was struck by an automobile. The initial assessment reveals that the patient is alert and oriented, is breathing, and has a carotid pulse. He has a wound on his right thigh that is spurting bright-red blood. You attempt to control the bleeding with direct pressure and elevation, but attempts are unsuccessful.
36. Based on the description, the bleeding is most likely:
    a. Venous
    b. Capillary
    c. Arterial
    d. Venule
37. Your next action for treating the patient is:
    a. Apply a tourniquet between the wound and heart.
    b. Apply a pressure point over the popliteal artery.
    c. Clamp the vessel with a hemostat.
    d. Apply a pressure point over the femoral artery.
38. If the previous action is *not* successful, then (and only then) you should:
    a. Apply a tourniquet between the wound and heart.
    b. Apply a pressure point over the popliteal artery.
    c. Clamp the vessel with a hemostat.
    d. Apply a pressure point over the femoral artery.

Questions 39 to 42 refer to the following scenario.
You respond to a call and find a 32-year-old woman who is the driver of a car involved in a front-end collision.

She is alert and oriented but appears pale and sweaty with delayed capillary refill; her neck veins are flat. She is complaining of pain in the upper-left quadrant of her abdomen and there are contusions on the left chest and abdominal walls. Her vital signs are respirations 26 breaths/min and shallow, pulse 120 beats/min and regular (at the carotids), and weak radial pulses. Her blood pressure is 70/50. Auscultation of her lungs reveals diminished breath sounds on the right side.

39. Based on these signs, what percentage of internal blood loss do you suspect has already occurred?
    a. Less than 10%
    b. 10% to 15%
    c. 20% to 25%
    d. More than 30%

40. The weak radial pulses in both arms are probably related to:
    a. Fractures
    b. Low blood pressure
    c. Blood clots
    d. Severed arteries in the arms

41. Based on these findings, which of the following oxygen delivery methods is appropriate?
    a. Venturi mask
    b. Nasal cannula
    c. Simple face mask
    d. Nonrebreather mask

42. If this patient had grossly distended neck veins, you would check for:
    a. Cardiac contusion
    b. Tension pneumothorax
    c. Aortic aneurysm
    d. Arrhythmias

Questions 43 to 45 refer to the following scenario.
You respond to a call and find a 30-year-old man who fainted after being robbed at gunpoint. His friend explains that the patient was unconscious for about 1 minute. The patient is now alert and oriented, and the physical examination is normal. His vital signs are pulse 80 beats/min and regular, blood pressure 100/80 mm Hg, and respirations 18 breaths/min and of normal depth.

43. This patient most likely has a transient form of:
    a. Obstructive shock
    b. Vasodilatory shock
    c. Hypovolemic shock
    d. Cardiogenic shock

44. What action should his friend have taken to facilitate the patient's recovery?
    a. Sit the patient up.
    b. Administer ammonia capsules.
    c. Elevate the legs while supine.
    d. Administer glucose by mouth.

45. This patient's primary cardiovascular problem was related to:
    a. A drop in blood pressure
    b. Tachycardia of the heart
    c. Vasoconstriction of the brain vessels
    d. Obstruction of blood flow through vessels

Questions 46 to 51 refer to the following scenario.
You respond to a call for a pedestrian struck by an automobile. You find a 50-year-old woman lying on her left side on the ground. Bystanders state that the patient was thrown approximately 30 feet after being struck by a car traveling at high speed. Your initial assessment of the patient reveals no response to verbal or painful stimuli, a shard of glass in her cheek protruding into her mouth with moderate bleeding, and gross deformity in both thighs. The patient also has a deep laceration to the medial aspect of her lower left leg with significant dark-red bleeding (not spurting). Vital signs are pulse 118 beats/min regular and weak, blood pressure 102/68 mm Hg, and respiratory rate 22 breaths/min and adequate.

46. Initial management of this patient's airway includes:
    a. Stabilizing the shard of glass in place.
    b. Maintaining the patient on her side and transporting rapidly.
    c. Removing the shard of glass and applying pressure to both sides of the laceration in the cheek.
    d. Stabilizing the shard of glass in place, positioning the patient supine, and suctioning as needed.

47. The appropriate position in which to transport this patient is:
    a. Prone
    b. Left lateral recumbent
    c. In the position she was found
    d. Supine

48. The bleeding in the leg is probably:
    a. Capillary bleeding
    b. Venous bleeding
    c. Arterial bleeding
    d. Caused by an underlying fracture

49. The first method to control the bleeding in the leg is by:
    a. Elevation
    b. Compression of the pressure point in the leg
    c. Application of a tourniquet
    d. Direct pressure

50. Attempts to control bleeding are not working and you decide to apply compression to a pressure point:
    a. Distal to the bleeding
    b. Proximal to the bleeding
    c. Directly over the wound
    d. Approximately 4 fingerbreadths below the injury

51. En route to the hospital you reevaluate the patient. The bleeding from her cheek and lower leg is controlled. Vital signs are pulse 138 beats/min and weak, blood pressure 72/40 mm Hg, and respiratory rate 24 breaths/min. At this stage the patient is demonstrating signs of:
    a. Decompensated shock
    b. Compensatory shock
    c. Obstructive shock
    d. Cardiogenic shock

119

21 Soft Tissue Injuries

MULTIPLE CHOICE

1. The surface or outermost layer of the skin is called the:
   a. Subcutaneous layer
   b. Fascia
   c. Epidermis
   d. Dermis

2. The special pigment in the epidermis that provides protection from the sun's radiation and contributes to skin color is called:
   a. Melanin
   b. Keratin
   c. Surfactant
   d. Sebum

3. When blood flow to the skin is reduced (as a result of vasoconstriction in hypovolemic shock or in cold temperatures), the skin may appear:
   a. Red
   b. Cyanotic
   c. Pale
   d. Mottled

4. The layer of skin that is composed of dense connective tissue that contains the nerves, blood vessels, sweat and sebaceous glands, and hair follicles is called the:
   a. Subcutaneous layer
   b. Fascia
   c. Epidermis
   d. Dermis

5. How is sensory perception affected if the dermis is completely damaged, as in a full-thickness burn?
   a. Increased sensory function
   b. Extreme pain
   c. No sensory function
   d. Tingling sensation

6. Beneath the skin is a layer of fat and connective tissue called the:
   a. Mucosa
   b. Subcutaneous layer
   c. Subdermal layer
   d. Peritoneum

7. In general, impaled objects should be:
   a. Stabilized in place
   b. Carefully removed
   c. Repositioned to facilitate bandaging
   d. Left alone

8. Objects impaled in the cheek should be:
   a. Stabilized in place
   b. Carefully removed
   c. Repositioned to facilitate bandaging
   d. Left alone

9. What vessels are likely to promote air embolism when severed?
   a. Arteries in head
   b. Veins in neck and upper chest
   c. Capillaries in chest
   d. Arteries in chest

10. When a neck vein is severed, you should:
    a. Apply a gauze dressing and sit the patient upright.
    b. Apply an airtight dressing and place the patient in the head-down position.
    c. Apply a saline dressing and place the patient on his or her side.
    d. Apply a multitrauma dressing and place the patient prone.

11. The first concern for a patient with injuries to the face and neck is the:
    a. Cervical spine
    b. Airway
    c. Eye
    d. Brain

12. Which of the following is a common effect of an improperly applied bandage?
    a. Obstruction of distal blood flow
    b. Damage to cartilage
    c. Obstruction of bowel function
    d. Tearing of muscles

13. The eye is a globular structure filled with gel-like fluid called the:
    a. Vitreous humor
    b. Mucus
    c. Peritoneal fluid
    d. Plasma

14. The collection of bones that surround the eye is called the:
    a. Ocular bones
    b. Orbit
    c. Periocular bones
    d. Acetabular

15. The white outer layer of the eye, which is composed of a tough, fibrous, and opaque protective membrane, is called the:
    a. Cornea
    b. Retina
    c. Lens
    d. Sclera

16. The pigmented or colored portion of the eye that regulates the diameter of the pupil is called the:
    a. Retina
    b. Iris
    c. Cornea
    d. Macula

121

17. Anatomically, the eye can be divided into anterior and posterior chambers by the:
    a. Lens
    b. Conjunctiva
    c. Retina
    d. Macula
18. When drainage of the aqueous humor is obstructed, eye pressure builds up and causes a condition known as:
    a. Retinitis
    b. Glaucoma
    c. Cataracts
    d. Aqueous tension
19. Tears are secreted from the:
    a. Mucous cells
    b. Ocular ducts
    c. Lacrimal glands
    d. Cornea
20. General principles for treating eye injuries include:
    a. Always irrigate and apply firm pressure.
    b. Avoid pressure and cover both eyes.
    c. Never treat in the field.
    d. Use petroleum gauze and never cover both eyes.
21. The best method in the field for removing foreign bodies of the eye is:
    a. With the use of suction cups
    b. Irrigation
    c. With the use of a cotton-tipped applicator
    d. With rapid eye movement
22. Impaled objects in the eyeball should be treated by:
    a. Pulling them out with a gloved hand.
    b. Repositioning them to facilitate bandaging.
    c. Stabilizing them in place.
    d. Leaving them alone.
23. Chemical burns to the eye are treated by:
    a. Bandaging the affected eye.
    b. Irrigating with water or sterile saline.
    c. Irrigating with an alkaline solution.
    d. Rapid transport without field treatment.
24. Light injuries caused by overexposure to infrared light from the sun or to ultraviolet light from arc welding are treated by:
    a. Placing moist patches over the eyes.
    b. Taping the eyes closed.
    c. Placing a cup over the eyes.
    d. Irrigating the eyes.
25. An extruded eyeball should be managed by:
    a. Replacing it in the eye socket.
    b. Covering it with dry 4 × 4 bandage and a patch.
    c. Covering it with a moist dressing and a cup.
    d. Irrigating during transport.
26. The outer visible flap of the ear is called the:
    a. Pinna
    b. Malleus
    c. Nares
    d. Vestibule
27. The middle ear communicates with the nasopharynx by the:
    a. Semicircular canal
    b. Cochlea
    c. Eustachian tube
    d. Vestibule
28. Other than hearing, the inner ear also contributes to control of:
    a. Voice transmission
    b. Heat exchange
    c. Balance and position
    d. Fluid exchange
29. Incomplete avulsed parts of the ear are treated by:
    a. Replacing them in anatomic position and bandaging them.
    b. Removing them and storing them in saline solution.
    c. Placing an ice pack over the site and transporting.
    d. Irrigating with Betadine and alcohol solution.
30. The rupture of the eardrum caused by changes in altitude and pressure is a type of:
    a. Tympanic syndrome
    b. Barotrauma
    c. The bends
    d. Pneumotympanic rupture
31. Amputated parts should be managed by:
    a. Placing them in a plastic bag and then placing the bag on ice.
    b. Soaking them in saline solution and placing them directly on ice.
    c. Wrapping them in an occlusive dressing to maintain moisture.
    d. Wrapping them in a multitrauma dressing to maintain sterility.
32. When applying a pressure bandage, you should use enough pressure to:
    a. Occlude distal flow.
    b. Cause venous distention.
    c. Cause tingling in the affected part.
    d. Control bleeding.
33. Skin that is blistered, red, blotchy, swollen, and very painful best describes a:
    a. Superficial or first-degree burn
    b. Partial-thickness or second-degree burn
    c. Full-thickness or third-degree burn
    d. Complete-thickness or fourth-degree burn
34. Which layer of the skin is injured in a superficial burn?
    a. Dermis
    b. Subcutaneous layer
    c. Epidermis
    d. Fascia
35. The most common cause of a superficial burn is:
    a. Scalding injury
    b. Sunburn
    c. Electrical injury
    d. Chemical injury

36. Which of the following burn types is likely to be most painful?
    a. Superficial
    b. Partial thickness
    c. Full thickness
    d. Fourth degree
37. Skin that appears charred, yellow brown, dark red, or white and translucent with thrombosed veins that are visible is probably related to a:
    a. Superficial burn
    b. Partial-thickness burn
    c. Full thickness burn
    d. Partial-thickness chemical burn
38. A major complication of circumferential burns completely around a body part (e.g., arm) is:
    a. Increased lactic acid production
    b. Obstructed blood flow to the part
    c. Increased heat to the cells beneath
    d. Killing of all superficial nerves
39. Which of the following body areas is considered critical when evaluating a burn patient?
    a. Armpits
    b. Scalp
    c. Groin (perineum)
    d. Thigh
40. Charring around the mouth and nose, black sputum, and singed nasal hairs and eyebrows are considered critical signs of:
    a. Respiratory burn injuries
    b. Eye injuries
    c. Chemical burn injuries
    d. Electrical injuries
41. The best dressing for a large thermal burn is:
    a. Petroleum gauze
    b. Dry sterile wrap
    c. Plastic wrap
    d. Moist sterile wrap
42. A common major complication of large surface area burns is:
    a. Cardiac arrhythmias
    b. Hypothermia
    c. Pulmonary embolus
    d. Bone infection
43. The most common cause of death from fires is:
    a. Fluid loss
    b. Infection
    c. Airway obstruction
    d. Smoke inhalation
44. The most common toxic gas that is inhaled in a fire is:
    a. Phosgene
    b. Carbon dioxide
    c. Carbon monoxide
    d. Cyanide
45. An early complication of direct heat transfer and burns to the respiratory tract is:
    a. Pulmonary fibrosis
    b. Bronchitis from mucus production
    c. Airway obstruction
    d. Pulmonary embolus

46. Carbon monoxide is a particularly toxic gas because it has a 200 times greater affinity than oxygen for:
    a. Diffusion
    b. Inhalation
    c. Hemoglobin
    d. Cell bonding
47. In burn patients, stridor and hoarseness may suggest:
    a. Bronchiolar injury
    b. Alveolar irritation
    c. Airway obstruction
    d. Nasal burns
48. In general, the most effective treatment for chemical burn injuries is:
    a. Application of cold packs on the affected area
    b. Irrigation with copious amounts of water
    c. Application of sterile dressing
    d. Application of gels to smother the burning process
49. Treatment of chemical burns requires:
    a. Application of a neutralizing agent
    b. Irrigation for 20 to 30 minutes
    c. Submersion in a small tub of water
    d. Rapid transport only
50. The force with which the movement of electrical current occurs is:
    a. Amperage
    b. Voltage
    c. Resistance
    d. Wattage
51. The number or volume of flowing electrons is called:
    a. Amperage
    b. Voltage
    c. Resistance
    d. Wattage
52. The degree of hindrance to electron flow is called:
    a. Amperage
    b. Voltage
    c. Resistance
    d. Wattage
53. Generally speaking, voltage:
    a. Causes more injury as it increases.
    b. Causes less injury as it increases.
    c. Does not affect the degree of injury.
    d. Cannot cause death when less than 60 cycles per second.
54. If electrical current passes through the brain, the primary complication is most likely:
    a. Cardiac arrest
    b. Cardiac arrhythmias
    c. Respiratory arrest
    d. Coronary thrombosis
55. Which of the following materials provides the greatest degree of resistance to electrical flow?
    a. Water
    b. Rubber
    c. Copper
    d. Steel

56. A large conducting body, such as the earth, that is used as a common return for an electrical circuit and an arbitrary zero of potential best describes:
    a. Current
    b. Voltage
    c. Flow
    d. Ground
57. The best action to take when a downed power line is in contact with the car you occupy is to:
    a. Step out of the car quickly.
    b. Step out of the car if you have rubber soles.
    c. Stay in the car until the power experts arrive.
    d. Step out of the car slowly.
58. What degree of resistance does wet skin provide to electricity?
    a. Low
    b. High
    c. Very high
    d. Zero
59. High voltage traveling through air and generating intense heat that can cause thermal burns is called a(n):
    a. Air burn
    b. Jump burn
    c. Light burn
    d. Arc burn
60. Which of the following is a complication of electrical current flowing through skeletal muscle?
    a. Fat tumors because of the release of lipoproteins
    b. Hyperglycemia from glucagon release
    c. Contractions preventing release of a grasped electrical source
    d. Explosion of the muscle and skin
61. Which type of burn is *not* included in estimating the extent of burn injury?
    a. First-degree burns
    b. Second-degree burns
    c. Third-degree burns
    d. Burns involving the bones, sometimes referred to as fourth-degree burns

MATCHING

Questions 62-66. Match the type of wound in column A with the description in column B.

Column A	Column B
62. _____ Contusion	a. Tearing away of skin's surface.
63. _____ Abrasion	b. Wound caused by sharp instrument driven through skin.
64. _____ Laceration	c. Scraping of skin surface or mucous membrane.
65. _____ Avulsion	d. Tearing of skin or other soft tissues.
66. _____ Puncture	e. Bruising of skin.

Questions 67-70. Match the type of bandage or dressing in column A with the description in column B.

Column A	Column B
67. _____ Multitrauma	a. Used as a sling or cravat bandage
68. _____ Triangular	b. Aluminum foil, plastic wrap, or petroleum gauze
69. _____ Self-adherent.	c. Large dressing used for massive abrasions or burns
70. _____ Occlusive	d. Allows elastic pressure for arterial bleeding

Questions 71-76. Match the correct percentage in column A with the burned body parts in column B.

Column A	Column B
71. _____ 27%	a. Infant's entire head.
72. _____ 36%	b. One leg and one arm of adult.
73. _____ 18%	c. Both arms (anterior and posterior) and anterior surface of both legs in adult.
74. _____ 9%	d. Entire anterior surface of adult.
75. _____ 46%	e. Both legs, groin, and one arm of adult.
76. _____ 50%	f. Adult's entire head.

FILL IN THE BLANK

Questions 77-83. List the following burn management steps in chronological order by assigning the numbers 1 through 5 to the treatment steps.

77. _____ Apply sterile dressing.

78. _____ Administer high-concentration oxygen.

79. _____ Open the airway.

80. _____ Remove rings and bracelets.

81. _____ Stop the burning process.

82. Generally, adults older than _____ years are considered at increased risk of burn severity.

83. Generally, children younger than _____ years are considered at increased risk of burn severity.

SHORT ANSWER

Questions 84-88. List five physical signs that should raise suspicion of inhalation injury.

84. _____

_____

85. _____

_____

86. _____

_____

87. _____

_____

88. _____

_____

CASE SCENARIOS

Questions 89 and 90 refer to the following scenario.
You find a 28-year-old man lying on the living room floor of his apartment and bleeding profusely from the face. His wife states that he tripped and fell on a glass coffee table. You note on examination that he is in severe respiratory distress and has a large fragment of glass impaled in his left cheek that projects into his oral cavity.

89. The greatest immediate risk with this patient is:
    a. Aspiration and airway obstruction
    b. Bleeding and death
    c. Neurogenic shock from panic
    d. Severe infection

90. Your first action for this patient should be to:
    a. Stabilize the glass with a stacked dressing and transport immediately.
    b. Turn the patient into the prone position and transport immediately.
    c. Remove the glass and hold direct pressure on the inside and outside of the wound.
    d. Place a suction catheter in the mouth and continuously suction during transport.

Questions 91 and 92 refer to the following scenario.
You respond to a construction site and find a 40-year-old worker in severe pain and holding his hand over his eye. Co-workers state that he was stabbed in the eye socket with a sharp pipe. On close examination you note that his left eye is completely avulsed and hanging approximately 3 inches out of the socket.

91. The immediate care of the eye should consist of:
    a. Dry 4 × 4 dressing
    b. Moist dressing
    c. Petroleum dressing
    d. Betadine-soaked dressing

92. After applying the dressing, the eyeball can be stabilized with:
    a. Adhesive tape
    b. A cup and bandage
    c. An elastic bandage
    d. A stacked bandage

Questions 93 to 95 refer to the following scenario.
A 14-year-old boy is found at the bottom of a stairwell with a large avulsion of the scalp. The 6-inch flap of skin is folded posteriorly, exposing a large area of subcutaneous tissue. It is attached to the remaining skin with a 1-inch segment of tissue. The patient is alert and oriented and has no disability finding, but you note clear liquid leaking from the ear.

93. The management of the avulsed part should include:
    a. Disconnecting the flap from the skin and storing it in a bag of ice.
    b. Rinsing the tissue and placing it in the normal anatomic position.
    c. Bandaging the flap as found with an elastic bandage.
    d. Placing an ice pack on the scalp and bandaging the flap in place.

94. The clear liquid leaking from the ear suggests a(n):
    a. Basilar skull fracture
    b. Eardrum rupture
    c. Wound infection
    d. Brainstem laceration

95. The leaking fluid should be managed by:
    a. Applying ice over the ear.
    b. Packing the ear with gauze.
    c. Applying a loose sterile dressing.
    d. Applying a cup over the ear.

Questions 96 and 97 refer to the following scenario.
A scuba diver complains of severe earache after descending to 50 feet below the surface. He states that he had a slight cold and congestion for 3 days before the dive.

96. Based on the history, what injury do you suspect?
    a. The bends
    b. Barotrauma to the eardrum
    c. Ruptured cochlea
    d. Severe middle ear infection

97. This problem is caused by a clogged:
    a. External ear
    b. Middle ear
    c. Eustachian tube
    d. Cochlea

Questions 98 to 100 refer to the following scenario.
You respond to a chemical manufacturing plant and find a 42-year-old woman who has received an entire body splash with an acid solution. She is alert and oriented and is in severe pain.

98. Your immediate action should be to:
    a. Provide rapid transport while irrigating with an intravenous solution en route.
    b. Have the patient remove all her clothing and place her in a shower to irrigate.
    c. Rinse the patient with an alkali solution to neutralize the acid.
    d. Irrigate with a mild acid solution (e.g., orange juice) to avoid a chemical reaction.

99. This patient's skin should be irrigated for a minimum of:
    a. 5 to 10 minutes
    b. 10 to 15 minutes
    c. 15 to 20 minutes
    d. 20 to 30 minutes

125

100. If this substance were a dry chemical, what actions would you take before irrigating?
    a. Neutralize the substance.
    b. Brush the substance off skin.
    c. Blow the substance off skin.
    d. Rub the substance off skin.

Questions 101 to 104 refer to the following scenario.
A 42-year-old man fell asleep while smoking in his den. His chair caught fire, and soon the house was in flames. The firefighters bring the man out of the burning house to your ambulance. The patient has blistering burns on his head and entire neck (completely around), anterior chest and abdomen, and groin. He has singed nasal hairs and eyebrows, and there is soot in the nostrils. His voice is very hoarse, and he is exhibiting stridor. He is alert, and his vital signs are respirations 20 breaths/min and regular, pulse 100 beats/min and regular, and blood pressure 140/70 mm Hg.

101. What percentage of this patient's body do you estimate is burned?
    a. 15%
    b. 21%
    c. 28%
    d. 35%
102. The burned areas are probably:
    a. Superficial
    b. Partial thickness
    c. Full thickness
    d. Fourth degree
103. What is your greatest concern regarding this patient?
    a. Hypovolemic shock from fluid loss
    b. Airway obstruction from respiratory burns
    c. Massive infection from surface area
    d. Neurogenic distributive shock from pain
104. How should oxygen be provided?
    a. By nasal cannula
    b. By high-concentration nonrebreather mask, humidified if possible
    c. By bag-mask
    d. By manually triggered resuscitator mask

Questions 105 to 108 refer to the following scenario.
You respond to a call and find a 2-year-old boy who has bitten into an electrical wire and appears to be having a grand mal seizure. His father is in a panic and is unable to provide a history of what happened. The child appears still to be biting the wire.

105. The child is probably still in contact with the wire because:
    a. He is having sustained contractions of the jaw.
    b. The wire had adhered to the mucosa.
    c. He has aspirated the wire into his pharynx.
    d. The wire has looped around his teeth.
106. Your immediate action would be to:
    a. Call the power company to disconnect the electricity.
    b. Find the fuse box and disconnect the fuse.
    c. Pull the plug from the outlet.
    d. Hit the child with a piece of wood to disconnect him from the wire.
107. Of the following, which offers the least resistance to electricity?
    a. Muscles
    b. Nerves
    c. Bone
    d. Fatty tissue
108. Once the child is disconnected from the wire, your first concern should be:
    a. Severe internal burns
    b. Destruction of the skeletal muscles
    c. Respiratory status
    d. Eye injuries from burns

109. Put the following steps for applying a bandage to the knee or elbow in proper sequential order.

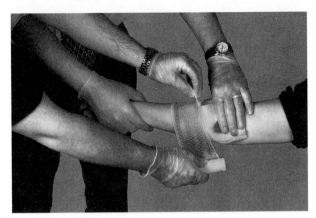

a. Start the roller bandage below the joint and anchor it in place.

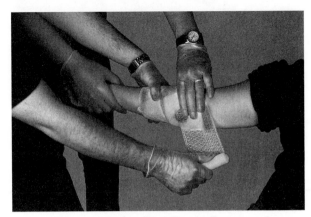

c. Traverse the bandage diagonally across the joint over the dressing.

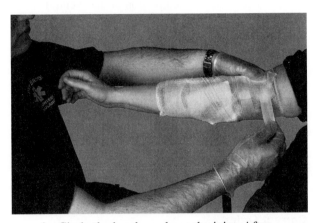

b. Circle the bandage above the joint. After circling the proximal portion, traverse downward to form an "X" over the dressing on the joint. Continue this pattern until the bandage is complete.

Correct Order

1. _____

2. _____

3. _____

Chapter **21** **Soft Tissue Injuries**

110. Put the following steps for removing a foreign body from the eye in proper sequential order.

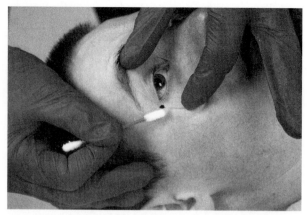

a. Gently whisk the foreign body off the eye with a clean, moistened cotton-tipped applicator.

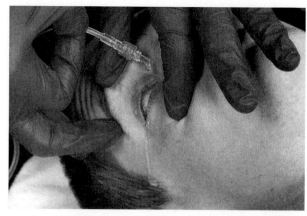

c. Allow a gentle stream of water to pass from the medial portion of the sclera over the rest of the eyeball as you attempt to flush away the foreign body. Respect the delicacy of the eyeball. Do not use a high-pressure stream. Rinse the affected portion of the eyelid if necessary.

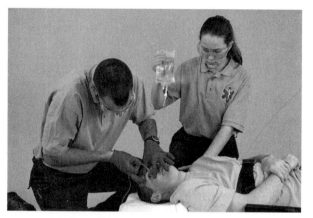

b. Use sterile water or saline or an intravenous administration set or a specially packaged eye-irrigating solution. Explain why you are taking the above actions to gain the patient's confidence and cooperation. This is especially important with children.

Correct Order

1. _____

2. _____

3. _____

22 Chest and Abdominal Trauma

Chest and Abdominal Trauma

MULTIPLE CHOICE

1. The thoracic cavity begins just below the neck and extends down to the:
   a. Umbilicus
   b. Pelvic girdle
   c. Diaphragm
   d. Xiphoid process
2. The total number of *pairs* of ribs is:
   a. 10
   b. 11
   c. 12
   d. 13
3. The lowest two pairs of ribs are called:
   a. Inferior ribs
   b. Floating ribs
   c. Thoracic ribs
   d. Superior ribs
4. The upper part of the sternum is called the:
   a. Manubrium
   b. Middle body
   c. Superior body
   d. Xiphoid process
5. During inspiration, the diaphragm:
   a. Relaxes and pushes downward into the abdomen.
   b. Contracts and pushes downward into the abdomen.
   c. Relaxes and rises into the thoracic cavity.
   d. Contracts and rises into the thoracic cavity.
6. During expiration, the diaphragm:
   a. Relaxes and pushes downward into the abdomen.
   b. Contracts and pushes downward into the abdomen.
   c. Relaxes and rises into the thoracic cavity.
   d. Contracts and rises into the thoracic cavity.
7. During forced exhalation, the upper portion of the right diaphragm can extend as high as the:
   a. Fourth costal cartilage anteriorly and to the eighth rib posteriorly
   b. Fourth costal cartilage anteriorly and to the tenth rib posteriorly
   c. Fifth costal cartilage anteriorly and to the eighth rib posteriorly
   d. Fifth costal cartilage anteriorly and to the tenth rib posteriorly
8. Which of the following structures are contained within the mediastinum?
   a. Heart, lungs, esophagus, and trachea
   b. Main stem bronchi, carotid arteries, heart, and lungs
   c. Heart, esophagus, main stem bronchus, and trachea
   d. Lungs, trachea, great vessels, and esophagus
9. The diaphragm connects to the ribs at what level?
   a. At the lower fifth pair of ribs
   b. At the lower sixth pair of ribs
   c. At the lower seventh pair of ribs
   d. At the lower eighth pair of ribs
10. The major cause of severe blunt trauma injury to the chest is:
    a. Falls
    b. Gunshot wounds
    c. Industrial accidents
    d. Motor vehicle crashes
11. Air in the pleural space is called a:
    a. Hydrothorax
    b. Hemothorax
    c. Pneumothorax
    d. Flail chest
12. Bleeding in the pleural space is called a:
    a. Hydrothorax
    b. Hemothorax
    c. Pneumothorax
    d. Flail chest
13. A flail portion of the chest wall is pulled inward by:
    a. Positive pressure during inhalation
    b. Positive pressure during exhalation
    c. Negative pressure during inhalation
    d. Negative pressure during exhalation
14. A patient presenting with severe swelling and ecchymosis of the neck and face after a heavy weight falling on his chest has:
    a. Cardiac tamponade
    b. Sucking chest wound
    c. Pneumothorax
    d. Traumatic asphyxia
15. A penetrating wound to the chest should be treated with:
    a. Supplemental oxygen and 4 × 4 gauze taped on three sides over wound
    b. Supplemental oxygen and 4 × 4 gauze taped on all four sides over wound
    c. Supplemental oxygen and occlusive dressing taped on three sides over wound
    d. Supplemental oxygen and occlusive dressing taped on all four sides over wound
16. Which organs are considered to be solid organs?
    a. Liver, spleen, and kidneys
    b. Stomach, pancreas, and liver
    c. Kidneys, bladder, and spleen
    d. Liver, bladder, and kidneys

17. The proper treatment for evisceration is:
   a. application of a dry, sterile dressing
   b. Replacing the intestines in the abdominal cavity
   c. application of a moist, sterile dressing
   d. pneumatic antishock garment

FILL IN THE BLANK

18. _____ _____ is the major vein that returns blood to the heart from the body.

19. _____ is the major artery that delivers blood from the heart to the body.

20. _____ is the "food pipe" that brings food from the mouth to the stomach.

21. _____ _____ is the lowest portion of the sternum.

22. The types of injury primarily responsible for tears of major vessels, especially the aorta, are

_____ _____.

23. The _____ peritoneum lines the abdominal and pelvic walls.

24. The _____ peritoneum covers most of the intraabdominal organs.

25. _____ is the term for inflammation of the peritoneum.

26. The abdomen is divided into quadrants by two

imaginary lines that intersect at the _____.

27. The pathway that allows pain to be localized anatomically near the affected organ is the

_____ pathway.

28. The presence of intestines protruding through a laceration in the abdominal wall is termed

_____.

29. Treatment of the patient with an acute abdomen

includes the administration of _____.

30. During the physical examination, you should begin

palpation _____ from the quadrant where the patient identifies the pain.

SHORT ANSWER

Questions 31-34. List four signs of a tension pneumothorax.

31. _____

32. _____

33. _____

34. _____

Questions 35 and 36. Identify the two distinct pathways by which abdominal pain may be transmitted.

35. _____

36. _____

Questions 37-39. List three common characteristics that the patient uses to describe visceral pain.

37. _____

38. _____

39. _____

Questions 40-47. During the focused (secondary) assessment, the chest and abdomen are examined for DCAP/BTLS. What does this mnemonic stand for?

40. D _____

41. C _____

42. A _____

43. P _____

44. B _____

45. T _____

46. L _____

47. S _____

Questions 48-51. List four possible findings that may be present in a patient who presents with an acute abdomen.

48. _____

130

Chapter **22** **Chest and Abdominal Trauma**

Copyright © 2010, 2007, 2004, 1997, 1992 by Mosby, Inc., an affiliate of Elsevier Inc. All rights reserved.

49. _____
   _____

50. _____
   _____

51. _____
   _____

TRUE/FALSE

52. _____ Penetrating gunshot wounds to the neck may cause severe chest injuries.
53. _____ The lower ribs protect the abdominal organs, and blunt trauma to the lower chest will not result in injury to these organs.
54. _____ A pneumothorax can be corrected in the field by positioning the patient supine with the legs elevated.
55. _____ A flail chest is when two or more ribs are broken in two or more places.
56. _____ A common cause of a flail chest is a gunshot wound.
57. _____ One method to stabilize a flail segment, in the patient without suspected neck or spinal injury, is to position the patient with the injured side down.
58. _____ A patient with cardiac tamponade will usually present with tracheal shift and distended neck veins.
59. _____ Blood in the mediastinum compresses the chambers of the heart in a patient with cardiac tamponade.
60. _____ An aortic tear is most common at the point where mobile and attached portions of the aorta meet.
61. _____ Eighty percent of patients with an aortic tear die at the scene.
62. _____ If a patient develops signs of a tension pneumothorax after an appropriate bandage has been applied to an open chest wound, you should immediately remove the dressing and reseal it after the release of the tension, which is at the end of a forced exhalation.
63. _____ Penetrating wounds to the lower chest cannot enter the abdominal cavity.
64. _____ The pelvic cavity is the lowermost portion of the abdominal cavity.
65. _____ Distention of the abdomen may not be apparent, even after significant abdominal bleeding.
66. _____ The primary goal of prehospital care for a patient with abdominal injuries is to summon advanced life support to the scene to stabilize the patient in the field.
67. _____ Blunt abdominal trauma may result from compression-type forces or from knife wounds.

68. _____ An injury to a hollow organ can often cause profuse bleeding, causing hypovolemic shock.
69. _____ A properly worn seat belt cannot cause deceleration force injuries on internal organs.

CASE SCENARIOS

Questions 70 to 74 are based on the following scenario.
You are called to the scene of a motor vehicle accident and find a patient behind the steering wheel complaining of chest pain and difficulty breathing. You notice that the airbag has deployed, but you "lift and look" and determine that the steering wheel has been deformed. The patient is alert and oriented, has significant bruising to the anterior chest wall, and has blood pressure of 90/62 mm Hg, pulse of 136 beats/min, respiratory rate of 32 breaths/min and shallow, and pale, cool, and moist skin. Your physical examination of the chest reveals a segment of the chest wall that is moving in the direction opposite the remaining chest wall, and there are diminished breath sounds on the left with normal breath sounds on the right.

70. Based on the chest wall movement, you suspect that this patient may have sustained a _____ _____ injury.
71. This physical finding, characterized by the segment of chest wall moving in the direction opposite the remaining chest wall, is termed _____ _____.
72. The breath sounds in the patient indicate the possible presence of _____ or _____.
73. You work with your partner and determine that the best method to use to extricate the patient from the car is the _____ _____.
74. The two major objectives in treating this patient's chest injury are _____ and _____.

Questions 75 to 78 are based on the following scenario.
You are called to the scene of a motor vehicle crash and find a 35-year-old woman who was the driver of the car lying supine next to the car. Bystanders inform you that the driver lost control of the car and went off the road and struck a tree at approximately 30 mph. You look in the car and identify that this older-model vehicle does not have an airbag. The patient was not wearing a seat belt. Your evaluation of the patient reveals a significant contusion on the chest wall consistent with striking the steering wheel. Your patient has a blood pressure of 82/60 mm Hg, heart rate of 132 beats/min, respiratory rate of 28 breaths/min, absent breath sounds on the right, good breath sounds on the left, distended neck veins, and the trachea shifted to the left.

131

75. Based on your evaluation of the patient, you suspect that the patient may have a:
    a. Pneumothorax
    b. Hemothorax
    c. Cardiac tamponade
    d. Tension pneumothorax
76. The best position to transport this patient is:
    a. Left lateral recumbent
    b. Supine with the head elevated
    c. Supine on a spine board with the neck and spine immobilized
    d. In the position of comfort

77. The tracheal shift in this patient is caused by:
    a. Blunt trauma to the neck
    b. Possible tension pneumothorax
    c. Possible pneumothorax
    d. Possible hemothorax
78. The distended neck veins are caused by the:
    a. Obstruction of blood returning to the heart through the large veins
    b. Obstruction of blood leaving the heart through the aorta
    c. Increased heart rate
    d. Patient's low blood pressure

CROSSWORD PUZZLE

Puzzle 22-1

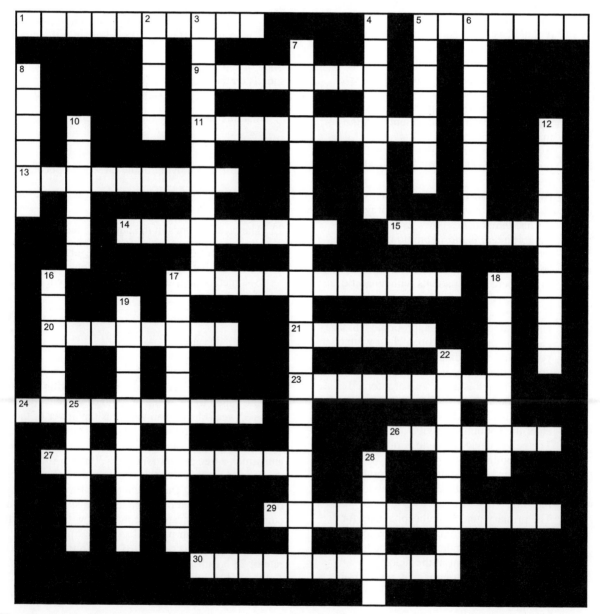

Across

1. _____ occurs when the diaphragm relaxes.
5. A _____ chest wound results from air drawn into the pleural space during inspiration.
9. Shoulder blades
11. Top of the ilium bone
13. The cavity bordered by the diaphragm and the pelvis
14. The reduced movement of the chest wall to avoid pain caused by broken or bruised ribs
15. _____ pneumothorax is a condition in which air entering the chest cavity cannot escape.
17. Collapse of a lung from air in the pleural space
20. Pain perceived in a location distant from the actual site
21. A single, large triangular bone of the pelvis
23. The uppermost portion of the sternum
24. Bleeding in the pleural space
26. The lowest portion of the sternum is called the _____ process.
27. Motor vehicle crashes are the major cause of severe _____ _____ to the chest.
29. Mechanism of injury that causes a tear of an organ or vessel from a point of attachment
30. The center of the thoracic cavity

Down

2. Major artery leaving the heart
3. _____ occurs when the diaphragm contracts.
4. Nerve pathway with imprecise perceptions to quality and location of pain
5. Nerve pathway perceiving clear quality of pain
6. Collarbones
7. Entrapment of air beneath the skin
8. Ribs are attached to the sternum by _____ cartilage.
10. Bruises to the flank are often associated with injuries to the _____.
12. Most common breath sound associated with pneumothorax
16. Protection is provided for the pelvic organs by the pelvic _____.
17. A sign of flail chest, exhibited by the opposing motion of the chest wall motion
18. Bony tip of the shoulder
19. Lining of the inner abdominal cavity
22. Respiratory muscle that separates the thorax and abdomen
25. Black or tarry stool
28. Cavity that is the lowermost portion of the abdomen

133

23 Musculoskeletal Care

MULTIPLE CHOICE

1. The axial skeleton consists of the:
   a. Skull, spine, ribs, and sternum
   b. Pelvis and lower extremities
   c. Upper extremities and clavicles
   d. The joints of the body

2. A softer precursor of bone that is present throughout the body and persists at sites of bone growth and at joints to provide a smooth, friction-free surface is called:
   a. Ligament
   b. Tendon
   c. Cartilage
   d. Fascia

3. Connective bands of tissue that attach bone to bone and maintain the stability of joints are called:
   a. Ligaments
   b. Tendons
   c. Cartilage
   d. Fascia

4. Thin bands of tissue that attach muscle to bone and initiate movement of joints are called:
   a. Ligaments
   b. Tendons
   c. Cartilage
   d. Fascia

5. The portion of bone responsible for the production of red blood cells is:
   a. Spongy bone
   b. Periosteum
   c. Bone marrow
   d. Epiphysis

6. The elbow is an example of a:
   a. Hinged joint
   b. Ball-and-socket joint
   c. Fused joint
   d. Gliding joint

7. Displacement of bones in a joint from their normal anatomic position is called a:
   a. Compression injury
   b. Dislocation
   c. Sprain
   d. Strain

8. The stretching or tearing of a ligament is called a:
   a. Compression injury
   b. Dislocation
   c. Sprain
   d. Strain

9. The term used to describe the sensation felt during palpation that is created by the grating of bone ends together is:
   a. Friction rub
   b. Homans' sign
   c. Rhonchi
   d. Crepitus

10. A joint locked in a deformed position after an injury is highly suggestive of a:
    a. Sprain
    b. Dislocation
    c. Strain
    d. Spiral fracture

11. The five Ps that may indicate vascular or nerve injury in a fractured extremity include pain, pulselessness, pallor, paresthesia (numbness or tingling), and:
    a. Paralysis
    b. Priapism
    c. Purple skin
    d. Palpitations

12. Bladder, rectal, and urethral injuries are often associated with fracture of the:
    a. Femur
    b. Lumbar spine
    c. Pelvis
    d. Hip

13. The most common sign or symptom of a fracture is:
    a. Discoloration
    b. Deformity
    c. Pain
    d. Swelling

14. Which of the following is a major cause of deformity after a fracture?
    a. The pulling force of opposing muscles
    b. Ecchymosis at the site of injury
    c. Obstruction of an artery
    d. Nerve paralysis in the extremity

15. Absence of capillary refill in a single extremity is highly suggestive of:
    a. Hypovolemic shock caused by severe blood loss and vasoconstriction
    b. Vascular compromise from a fracture or dislocation
    c. Spinal shock causing vasoconstriction to one side of the body
    d. Cardiac tamponade causing poor cardiac output through the aorta

16. A primary rule of fracture management is to splint the fracture site and the:
   a. Surrounding tissues
   b. Distal extremity
   c. Adjacent joints
   d. Proximal extremity
17. The bone that can be palpated on the anterior upper chest region that extends from the sternum to the shoulder region is called the:
   a. Scapula
   b. Glenoid
   c. Olecranon
   d. Clavicle
18. Injuries to the shoulder, humerus, scapula, and clavicle are best treated with a(n)
   a. Pillow splint
   b. Sling and swathe
   c. Rigid splint
   d. Air splint
19. The most common mechanism of injury for the upper extremity is a:
   a. Direct blow
   b. Fall on an outstretched hand
   c. Twisting force
   d. Hyperextension injury
20. Shoulder dislocations are frequently caused by a:
   a. Blow to the scapula
   b. Fall on an outstretched arm
   c. Tugging force applied to the arm
   d. Blow to the clavicle
21. Vascular compromise resulting from shoulder dislocations can be evaluated by palpating the:
   a. Popliteal artery
   b. Dorsalis pedis artery
   c. Radial artery
   d. Humeral artery
22. The longest and strongest bone of the body is the:
   a. Humerus
   b. Tibia
   c. Fibula
   d. Femur
23. A patient who has an extremity with a good pulse with no feeling or movement has probably injured a(n):
   a. Ligament
   b. Growth plate
   c. Artery
   d. Nerve
24. Angulated elbow fractures or dislocations are best immobilized by a(n):
   a. Pillow splint on medial side of arm
   b. Sling and swathe
   c. Rigid splint, with sling and swathe
   d. Air splint extending from wrist to axilla
25. The bones of the forearm include the radius and the:
   a. Humerus
   b. Fibula
   c. Manubrium
   d. Ulna

26. Using the basic rules of splinting, fractures of the wrist should be immobilized from the finger to the:
   a. Midforearm
   b. Wrist
   c. Shoulder
   d. Humerus
27. Placing a roller bandage in the hand before splinting fractures places the hand in the position of:
   a. Extension
   b. Rotation
   c. Function
   d. Articulation
28. Multiple fractures of the pelvis associated with hypovolemic shock are best treated by:
   a. A traction splint
   b. Pneumatic antishock garment (PASG)
   c. Rigid 3- and 5-foot splints
   d. Tying the legs together
29. The lower leg bone that can be palpated on the anterior lower leg is the:
   a. Fibula
   b. Radius
   c. Tibia
   d. Talus
30. Which of the following fractures is often associated with spinal injuries?
   a. Patella
   b. Calcaneus
   c. Metatarsal
   d. Hip
31. Pelvic fractures in stable patients are best splinted by:
   a. Rigid 3- and 5-foot splints
   b. Securing patient to long spine board
   c. Traction splint application
   d. PASG application

MATCHING

Questions 32-34. Match the appropriate muscle in column A with the structures in column B.

Column A		Column B
32. _____ Smooth		a. Blood vessel
33. _____ Cardiac		b. Biceps
34. _____ Skeletal		c. Heart

Questions 35-37. Match the appropriate mechanism of injury in column A with the type of force in column B.

Column A	Column B
35. _____ Bumper striking tibia, causing transverse fracture at site of impact.	a. Twisting force b. Indirect force along bone's axis c. Direct force
36. _____ Ice skater fracturing tibia during spin when blade stuck in ice.	
37. _____ Humerus fracture after fall on outstretched hand.	

Questions 38-42. Match the description in column A with the type of splint in column B.

Column A

38. _____ Made of padded cardboard, wood, metal, or plastic.
39. _____ Environmental temperature can impair function.
40. _____ Best splint for femur fracture.
41. _____ Best ankle splint.
42. _____ Can be made from triangular bandages.

Column B

a. Traction splint
b. Pillow splint
c. Rigid splint
d. Sling and swathe
e. Air splint

Questions 43-48. Match the fracture or dislocation in column A with the splinting method in Column B.

Column A

43. _____ Dislocated shoulder
44. _____ Fractured ankle
45. _____ Fractured hand
46. _____ Fractured tibia
47. _____ Fractured finger
48. _____ Fractured femur

Column B

a. Traction splint
b. 3- and 5-foot splints
c. Sling and swathe
d. Tongue blade splint
e. Pillow splint
f. Rigid 9-inch splint

FILL IN THE BLANK

49. Numbness or tingling is also called _____.
50. When applying the Sager traction splint, mechanical traction should be applied by using _____% of the patient's body weight, not to exceed _____ pounds of traction.
51. When applying a Hare traction splint, the _____ strap should be applied first.
52. When applying a splint that encompasses the hand, the hand should be splinted in the _____.
53. The _____ is the major weight-bearing bone of the lower leg.

SHORT ANSWER

Questions 54 and 55. List the two goals of management for patients with extremity injuries.

54. _____
_____

55. _____
_____

Questions 56-59. List the four signs and symptoms of nerve injury.

56. _____
_____

57. _____
_____

58. _____
_____

59. _____
_____

CASE SCENARIOS

Questions 60 to 62 refer to the following scenario.
You respond to a call and find an 83-year-old woman complaining of pain in the midthigh region. She states that she fell from a ladder and landed on her foot and heel. The leg feels quite stable, and she is able to walk on it.

60. Based on the history, what type of fracture is this patient most likely to have sustained?
   a. Stable femur fracture
   b. Open femur fracture
   c. Dislocated hip
   d. Fractured hip
61. The mechanism of injury for this patient is best described as:
   a. Direct
   b. Twisting
   c. Indirect
   d. Rotational
62. The splint of choice for this patient is:
   a. Traction
   b. Pillow
   c. 3-inch lateral splints
   d. Long spine board

Questions 63 to 65 refer to the following scenario.
You respond to a call and find a 24-year-old ice skater who fell on an outstretched arm and is complaining of shoulder pain. She is supporting her forearm with her opposite hand, and her upper arm is positioned slightly away from her chest wall on the injured side. You note deformity and tenderness in the shoulder region.

63. Based on the history and physical examination, you suspect a(n):
   a. Fracture shaft of the humerus
   b. Anterior shoulder dislocation
   c. Fracture of the scapula
   d. Fracture of the olecranon
64. The splint of choice for this patient is a(n):
   a. Rigid board splint
   b. Air splint
   c. Pillow splint
   d. Sling and swathe
65. Given the site and nature of this injury, what complication are you most concerned about in this patient?
   a. Hemorrhage at the site of injury
   b. Fat embolism
   c. Neurovascular compromise
   d. Poor healing

137

Questions 66 to 68 refer to the following scenario.
You respond to a call and find a 74-year-old man
complaining of hip pain. He states that he simply
stepped off a high curb and planted his foot forcefully
on the ground and felt severe pain in his hip. He is lying
on the ground, and his leg appears externally rotated
and shortened.

66. Based on the history and physical examination, you
    suspect a:
    a. Minor muscle injury
    b. Dislocation of the hip
    c. Fracture of the hip
    d. Pelvic fracture

67. Given the minor nature of the mechanism of injury,
    what preexisting condition might explain this
    injury?
    a. Osteoporosis
    b. Arteriosclerosis
    c. Hypercalcemia
    d. Stress injury

68. The best method to transport this patient will be:
    a. Prone on the ambulance stretcher
    b. In the left lateral recumbent position
    c. Supine with knees flexed
    d. Supine on a long back board with the patient
       secured to the board

Questions 69 to 71 refer to the following scenario.
A 45-year-old construction worker fell from a 20-foot
scaffold and landed on his feet. He is found lying on his
left side. He is pale, sweaty, and has delayed capillary
refill. His blood pressure is 80/60 mm Hg, and his pulse
is 140 beats/min and regular. You note that his left leg is
deformed at the midthigh region and at the middle
lower leg. His right leg appears normal, but he has no
dorsalis pedis or posterior tibial pulses in either leg.

69. Based on the history and physical examination,
    your immediate concern is:
    a. Losing the extremities because of poor blood
       supply
    b. Decompensated hypovolemic shock
    c. Causing open fractures during transport
    d. Paralysis of the right leg

70. The absence of pulses in both legs is probably
    related to:
    a. The vasoconstriction response of shock
    b. Compression of an artery because of fractures
    c. Swelling in the thighs
    d. Peripheral nerve injury

71. Treatment for this patient includes:
    a. Spinal immobilization and high-concentration
       oxygen
    b. Application of the PASG with inflation of the
       abdominal section only
    c. High-concentration oxygen and securing the
       patient to the long board in the left lateral
       recumbent position
    d. Rapid transport with the neck immobilized in a
       cervical collar and the patient positioned supine
       on the stretcher with his head elevated

Questions 72 and 73 refer to the following scenario.
A 40-year-old female pedestrian is struck in the left
knee region by an automobile. You note the leg is
grossly angulated at the left knee, and pulses are absent
on the injured side. The patient also has a deformity in
her right wrist. Otherwise the patient is stable and has
no other obvious injuries.

72. Based on these findings, you should:
    a. Splint the leg as you found it.
    b. Attempt gentle straightening to regain pulse.
    c. Apply traction with a hare or Sager splint.
    d. Elevate the limb in the angulated position.

73. The hand and wrist should be placed in the position
    of function and splinted with a:
    a. Traction splint
    b. Rigid splint
    c. Pillow splint
    d. Sling and swathe

Puzzle 23-1

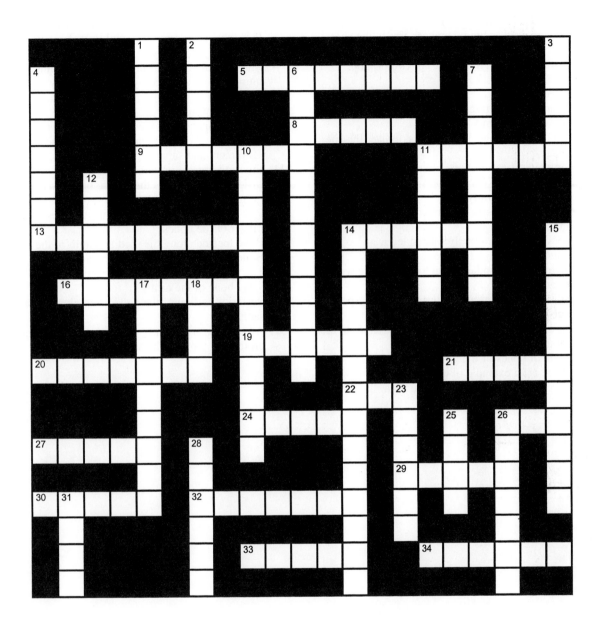

Across

5. Force usually transmitted along the axis of bone
8. _____ splints are made of cardboard, wood, metal, or plastic.
9. Ankle bones
11. A bandage used to bind the upper arm to the chest wall
13. Serves as a cushion at the sites of two or more bones
14. Injury to ligaments
16. An open or _____ fracture communicates with the outside environment.
19. A _____ fracture has no break in skin over the site.
20. Kneecap
21. Major weight-bearing bone of the lower leg
22. Pneumatic or _____ splints provide circumferential support to an extremity.
24. Skeleton that supports and protects the internal organs
26. A shortened and externally rotated leg is an indication of a _____ fracture.
27. Triangle-shaped bandage used to support the weight of the arm
29. Winglike bone forming the superior lateral aspect of the pelvis
30. Calcified connective tissues that give strength to the skeleton
32. Eight small bones of the wrist
33. The knee is an example of a _____ joint.
34. Long bone that runs parallel to the tibia

Down

1. Involuntary or _____ muscles contract automatically and are not under the individual's control.
2. Longest and strongest bone in the body
3. Pain, abnormal sensation, and loss of movement are signs of _____ injury.
4. Muscle that is similar in structure to voluntary muscle but is directed by the involuntary nervous system
6. To flex upward
7. Tough connective tissue that binds bone to bone
10. The _____ skeleton is primarily concerned with movement and support of the erect body.
11. Injury to muscle or tendon
12. Inside of bone that is the source of blood cells
14. Framework of the body
15. Five bones from the wrist to the knuckles
17. Finger or toe bones
18. Bone located along the medial length of the forearm
23. Bone on the lateral aspect of the arm
25. The most common symptom of bone or joint injury
26. Long bone of the arm
28. Posterior portion of the pelvic ring along with the sacrum
31. An obvious sign of an _____ fracture is a bone protruding through the skin.

24 Injuries to the Head and Spine

MULTIPLE CHOICE

1. The nervous system is structurally divided into two main divisions: the central nervous system and the:
   a. Peripheral nervous system
   b. Ganglionic nervous system
   c. Proximal nervous system
   d. Core nervous system

2. The central nervous system is made up of the brain, the brainstem, and the:
   a. Afferent nerves
   b. Peripheral nerves
   c. Dermatomes
   d. Spinal cord

3. The nervous system can also be divided by function, creating the voluntary division and:
   a. Paravoluntary division
   b. Autonomic division
   c. Reflex division
   d. Ganglionic division

4. Willful activities such as running to catch a train, reaching for an object, or buttoning a shirt are examples of functions mediated through the:
   a. Autonomic division
   b. Reflex division
   c. Spinal division
   d. Voluntary division

5. The control of the heart, the glands, and smooth muscles within organs such as the digestive tract is mediated through the:
   a. Autonomic division
   b. Reflex division
   c. Spinal division
   d. Voluntary division

6. There are two main divisions of the autonomic nervous system: the parasympathetic and the:
   a. Paraspinal
   b. Parasympathomimetic
   c. Sympathetic
   d. Sympathomimetic

7. Which of the following is mediated through the parasympathetic nervous system?
   a. Sweating
   b. Constriction of pupils
   c. Increasing the heart rate
   d. Vasoconstriction

8. If complete cessation of oxygen delivery occurs, as in cardiac arrest, the patient will become unconscious in about:
   a. 5 seconds
   b. 1 minute
   c. 4 to 6 minutes
   d. 10 minutes

9. Approximately how long will it take for irreversible brain damage to occur when the brain is totally deprived of oxygen?
   a. 5 to 10 seconds
   b. 1 to 2 minutes
   c. 2 to 3 minutes
   d. 4 to 6 minutes

10. The most sensitive indicator of inadequate oxygenation of the brain is:
    a. Alteration in mental status
    b. Motor function
    c. Sensory function
    d. Heart rate

11. The brainstem exits the lower skull through an opening called the:
    a. Foramen arteriosum
    b. Foramen magnum
    c. Foramen ovale
    d. Foramen minor

12. The space within the adult cranium has a capacity of about:
    a. 0.5 L
    b. 1.0 L
    c. 2.0 L
    d. 3.0 L

13. If the pressure within the cranium becomes severe, the brain may be forced down through the opening in the base of the skull. This dire emergency is called:
    a. Displacement
    b. Herniation
    c. Pressure syndrome
    d. Compression syndrome

14. Most vertebrae are held together by ligaments and separated by:
    a. Disks
    b. Nerves
    c. Bone
    d. Tendons

15. The three-layered membranous coverings of the brain and spinal cord that serve to protect the central nervous system are called the:
    a. Pleura
    b. Periosteum
    c. Myelin sheath
    d. Meninges

16. The largest and most superior portion of the brain is called the:
    a. Cerebrum
    b. Brainstem
    c. Cerebellum
    d. Diencephalon

141

17. The lower part of the brain consisting of bundles and tracts of nerves traveling down to the spinal cord and with distinct nerve cell centers of its own is called the:
    a. Cerebrum
    b. Brainstem
    c. Cerebellum
    d. Diencephalon
18. The posterior outpocketing of the brain that is primarily concerned with coordination of movement and balance is called the:
    a. Cerebrum
    b. Brainstem
    c. Cerebellum
    d. Diencephalon
19. Injuries that cause disruption of specific sections of brain tissue or nerves (e.g., gunshot wounds) and result in loss of specific functions are called:
    a. Metabolic
    b. Secondary
    c. Structural
    d. Contained
20. Problems that affect all the brain cells equally, such as hypoxia, low blood sugar, shock, and poisoning, are called:
    a. Metabolic
    b. Secondary
    c. Structural
    d. Contained
21. Hypoxia, hypotension, hypoglycemia, infections, and increased intracranial pressure are examples of:
    a. Secondary brain injuries
    b. Primary brain injuries
    c. Modifying brain injuries
    d. Complicating brain injuries
22. Injuries that occur on the opposite side of the brain from the site of the blow (from dynamic movement of brain after initial impact) are called:
    a. Compression injuries
    b. Deceleration injuries
    c. Contrecoup injuries
    d. Ipsilateral contusions
23. Cerebrospinal fluid leaking from the ear should be treated by:
    a. Packing the ear to contain fluid.
    b. Attaching a loose, sterile dressing over the ear.
    c. Doing nothing.
    d. Placing the patient on the affected side.
24. Raccoon eyes, Battle's sign, and cerebrospinal fluid leakage from the nose or ear are signs of:
    a. Brain laceration
    b. Epidural hematoma
    c. Basilar skull fracture
    d. Increased intracranial pressure
25. A transient loss of consciousness or neurologic function from a blow to the brain is called a:
    a. Contusion
    b. Concussion
    c. Compression
    d. Contortion

26. Headaches, nausea, and vomiting (sometimes projectile) are common signs of:
    a. Skull fracture
    b. Brain contusion
    c. Increased intracranial pressure
    d. Infection
27. Which of the following vital sign presentations may signify increased intracranial pressure?
    a. Decreased pulse rate, increased blood pressure
    b. Increased pulse rate, decreased blood pressure
    c. Decreased pulse rate, decreased blood pressure
    d. Increased pulse rate, increased blood pressure
28. Epidural hematomas are caused by:
    a. Arterial bleeding
    b. Capillary bleeding
    c. Venous bleeding
    d. Venule bleeding
29. Subdural hematomas are caused by:
    a. Arterial bleeding
    b. Capillary bleeding
    c. Venous bleeding
    d. Venule bleeding
30. The manual airway maneuver of choice for the head-injured patient is:
    a. Head-tilt/chin-lift
    b. Head-tilt/neck-lift
    c. Jaw thrust without head tilt
    d. Triple airway maneuver
31. What is the effect of increased carbon dioxide level on cerebral vessels?
    a. Constriction
    b. Dilation
    c. Spasm
    d. Obstruction
32. The Glasgow Coma Scale score for a patient who has no verbalizations, does not open the eyes, and is decorticate (has abnormal flexion) to painful stimuli is:
    a. 4
    b. 5
    c. 7
    d. 9
33. The first priority in the management of a patient with a severe head trauma is:
    a. Performing a neurologic examination.
    b. Establishing an airway and adequate ventilation.
    c. Applying a cervical collar.
    d. Controlling bleeding from the scalp.
34. When the spinal cord is injured at a low cervical level (C7) or a high thoracic level (T1), the respiratory function is most likely to be:
    a. Respiratory arrest
    b. Intercostal breathing only
    c. Diaphragmatic breathing only
    d. Normal respiration

35. When the spinal cord is injured at a high cervical level (C2), the respiratory function is most likely to be:
    a. Respiratory arrest
    b. Intercostal breathing only
    c. Diaphragmatic breathing only
    d. Normal respiration

36. When a patient develops neurogenic shock from spinal injuries, the pulse rate is most likely to be:
    a. Slow (below 60)
    b. Normal range (60-80)
    c. Fast (above 100)
    d. Very fast (above 150)

37. The vessels of a patient in neurogenic shock are most likely to be:
    a. Constricted
    b. Dilated
    c. Normal
    d. Collapsed

38. The loss of sympathetic tone of a patient in neurogenic shock may result in penile erection, which is called:
    a. Neuroerection
    b. Priapism
    c. Sympathetic erection
    d. Penile dilation

39. The most common cause of spinal cord injury is:
    a. Motor vehicle crashes
    b. Falls
    c. Sports-related incidents
    d. Diving incidents

40. The most common sites of vertebral injury are where vertebrae that allow motion meet:
    a. The rib cage
    b. Vertebrae that are fixed
    c. Other mobile vertebrae
    d. Intervertebral disks

41. The term used to describe a hyperextension injury resulting from a rear-end collision is:
    a. Contrecoup
    b. Whiplash
    c. Posterior extension
    d. Subluxation

42. When immobilizing a spinal injury patient, you should *not* return the neck to the neutral position if:
    a. The neck is flexed.
    b. Resistance is encountered.
    c. The neck is extended.
    d. Contusions are noted on the neck.

43. Which of the following characteristics are typical of a sports helmet but not a motorcycle helmet?
    a. Easier access to the airway
    b. Should always be removed
    c. Has a Plexiglas face shield
    d. Should never be removed

44. During the initial step of spinal immobilization when removing a helmet, the head is stabilized by holding:
    a. Only the helmet
    b. Only the mandible
    c. Both the helmet and the mandible
    d. Only the maxilla

MATCHING

Questions 45-49. Match the bones in column A with the related region of the skull in column B. You can use the column B selections more than once.

Column A	Column B
45. _____ Mandible	a. Cranium
46. _____ Parietal	b. Face
47. _____ Maxilla	
48. _____ Temporal	
49. _____ Occipital	

Questions 50-54. Match the type of vertebrae in column A with the number of vertebrae in column B.

Column A	Column B
50. _____ Cervical	a. 5 (mobile)
51. _____ Lumbar	b. 4 (fused)
52. _____ Coccyx	c. 12
53. _____ Sacral	d. 5 (fused)
54. _____ Thoracic	e. 7

Questions 55-57. Match the appropriate membranous layer in column A with the description in column B.

Column A	Column B
55. _____ Pia mater	a. Tough, leathery outer layer
56. _____ Arachnoid	b. Middle layer
57. _____ Dura mater	c. Inner layer

Questions 58-60. Match the category in column A with the type of action mediated by the central nervous system in column B.

Column A	Column B
58. _____ Automatic	a. Withdrawal from hot candle
59. _____ Reflex	b. Breathing, heart rate, etc
60. _____ Conscious	c. Lifting a box

Questions 61-65. Match the area of the brain in column A with its functions in column B.

Column A	Column B
61. _____ Frontal lobe	a. Vision
62. _____ Parietal lobe	b. Intelligence, motor function
63. _____ Occipital lobe	c. Respiratory function
64. _____ Brainstem	d. Sensory function
65. _____ Temporal lobe	e. Hearing, smell

Questions 66 and 67. Match the type of skull fracture in column A with the description in column B.

Column A

66. _____ Basilar
67. _____ Depressed

Column B

a. Crack in floor of skull
b. Bone fragments pressed downward toward brain

Questions 68-71. Match the appropriate spinal nerve level in column A with the anatomic sensory area (dermatome) in column B.

Column A

68. _____ Fourth thoracic (T4)
69. _____ Fourth cervical (C4)
70. _____ First lumbar (L1)
71. _____ Tenth thoracic (T10)

Column B

a. Groin
b. Nipple
c. Above clavicle
d. Umbilicus

Questions 72-74. Match the type of spinal injury force in column A with the mechanisms of injury in column B.

Column A

72. _____ Compression
73. _____ Flexion
74. _____ Extension

Column B

a. Face striking windshield in a front-end collision
b. Occipital region striking bottom of pool during a dive
c. Top portion of skull striking bottom of pool during a dive

Questions 75-77. Match the approach to immobilization in column A to the situation in column B.

Column A

75. _____ Short board
76. _____ Long board
77. _____ Rapid extrication

Column B

a. Unstable driver of a car
b. Pedestrian struck by car
c. Stable driver of a car

Questions 78-80. Match the circumstances in column A with removing or not removing the helmet in column B.

Column A

78. _____ Good fit with little or no movement.
79. _____ Inability to access airway.
80. _____ Proper spinal immobilization cannot be performed in place.

Column B

a. Remove helmet
b. Do not remove helmet

FILL IN THE BLANK

81. _____ _____ is the fluid that surrounds the brain and offers some protection to it.

82. _____ is the color of the fluid that surrounds the brain.

83. _____ is the term for the soft spots present in the top of the skull during infancy.

84. The common term _____ _____ used for ecchymosis around the eyes, is a sign of a fracture at the base of the skull.

85. The _____ _____ _____ is the artery located on the inside surface of the temporal bone and may be a cause of significant bleeding if this area of the skull is fractured.

86. A period of memory loss is called _____.

TRUE/FALSE

87. _____ During hypoventilation the carbon dioxide level in the blood decreases.

88. _____ If you reduce the carbon dioxide content of the blood, the blood flow to the head will also be reduced.

89. _____ Patients who are being immobilized on a long spine board should have the head secured to the board before the torso.

90. _____ If you need to remove a football helmet to properly manage the patient's airway, the shoulder pads should also be removed.

91. _____ Classically, a subdural hematoma presents with a short period of unconsciousness, followed by a lucid interval and then a decrease or alteration in the patient's level of consciousness.

CASE SCENARIOS

Questions 92 and 93 refer to the following scenario.
A 25-year-old unconscious man was involved in a motor vehicle crash. Bystanders state that he was initially unconscious, became conscious 3 minutes after the crash, and lapsed into unconsciousness again about 5 minutes ago. He is unresponsive to pain. Physical assessment reveals left pupil dilated and nonreactive; blood pressure 200/110 mm Hg, pulse 42 beats/min and bounding, and respirations irregular at an approximate rate of 8 breaths/min. He has a contusion and crepitus in the temporal region of the skull.

92. What do you suspect is this patient's major underlying problem?
   a. Brain contusion
   b. Epidural hematoma
   c. Concussion
   d. Subarachnoid hemorrhage

93. What is the likely cause of the change in this patient's vital signs?
   a. Increased intracranial pressure
   b. Direct injury to the brain
   c. The age of the patient
   d. A history of hypertension

Questions 94 to 99 refer to the following scenario.
A 14-year-old falls approximately 7 feet from a swing and strikes his left forehead on a soft rubber mat, knocking him unconscious. After 30 seconds, he awakes

and says he feels "all right." You find the youngster alert and breathing 24 times per minute with his abdominal muscles only. Vital signs are pulse 68 beats/min and regular and blood pressure 76/60 mm Hg. He cannot move his arms and legs and has sensation above the clavicle but none at nipple line. You also note priapism.

94. Based on the presenting signs, you suspect spinal injury at the level of the:
    a. High thoracic or low cervical spine
    b. Low thoracic or high lumbar spine
    c. High cervical spine
    d. Low lumbar or high sacral spine
95. Based on the vital signs, what complication do you suspect?
    a. Increased intracranial pressure
    b. Neurogenic (spinal) shock
    c. Obstructive shock
    d. Epidural hematoma
96. The vital signs, priapism, and loss of the sweat mechanism below the clavicles are a result of:
    a. Increased parasympathetic activity
    b. Increased sympathetic activity
    c. Decreased parasympathetic activity
    d. Decreased sympathetic activity
97. His respiratory status is caused by a loss of:
    a. Diaphragm function
    b. Intercostal muscle function
    c. Abdominal muscle function
    d. Neck muscle function
98. The initial loss of consciousness is probably caused by a(n):
    a. Contusion
    b. Laceration
    c. Concussion
    d. Epidural bleed
99. Treatment of this patient should include spinal immobilization and:
    a. Oxygen by nonrebreather mask
    b. Oxygen by nasal cannula
    c. Oxygen by Venturi mask
    d. No oxygen

Questions 100 to 103 refer to the following scenario.
A 40-year-old man was in a front-end auto collision and lost consciousness. When the ambulance arrived, the patient refused medical evaluation and treatment. A week later, the man became unconscious while watching television at home. On your arrival on the scene, the patient is unresponsive to painful stimuli. His vital signs are blood pressure 150/100 mm Hg, respirations 28 breaths/min and very deep, and pulse 80 beats/min. His left pupil is fixed and dilated, and his right pupil is midpositional with normal reactivity.

100. Based on the history and presenting signs, what do you think is the primary problem?
    a. Cerebral contusion
    b. Stroke
    c. Subdural hematoma
    d. Subarachnoid hemorrhage
101. The bleeding within the skull is most likely:
    a. Arterial
    b. Capillary
    c. Venous
    d. Arteriole
102. The initial loss of consciousness after the crash was probably caused by a(n):
    a. Concussion
    b. Contusion
    c. Laceration
    d. Abrasion
103. Based on the ventilatory status, what approach would you use to deliver oxygen?
    a. Nasal cannula
    b. Nonrebreather mask
    c. Bag-mask
    d. Simple face mask

145

104. Put in proper sequential order the following steps for placing a patient in supine position on a long spine board using the log roll.

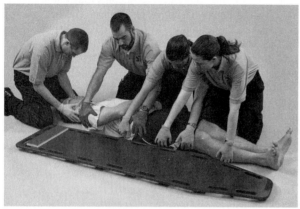

a. Three EMTs are positioned at the patient's side at the level of the chest, hips, and lower extremities while the long spine board is positioned on the other side of the patient. Check the patient's arm on the side of the EMTs for injury before log-rolling the patient. Align the lower extremities.

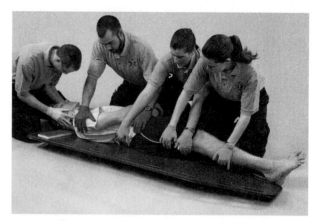

c. On command from the EMT at the head, the EMTs gently roll the patient onto the board, then roll the board to the ground.

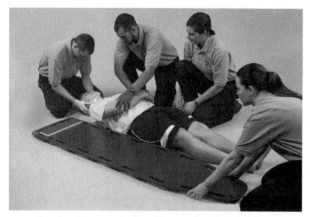

b. Apply a cervical collar, and place the patient's arms by his or her side or across the chest. One EMT maintains manual cervical stabilization throughout the procedure.

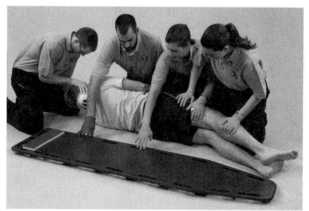

d. On command from the EMT at the head, all EMTs should rotate the patient toward themselves, keeping the body in alignment. The EMTs then reach across with one hand and pull the board toward the patient.

146

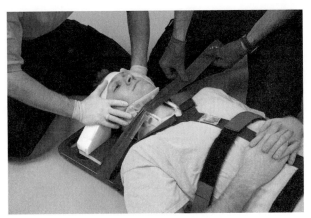

e. Immobilize the head with a head immobilizer or tape.

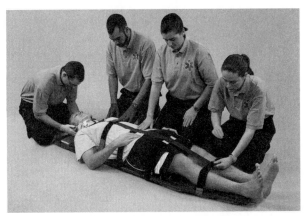

f. Strap the patient's torso and extremities securely to the board.

Correct Order

1. _____

2. _____

3. _____

4. _____

5. _____

6. _____

Chapter **24 Injuries to the Head and Spine**

25 Infants and Children

MULTIPLE CHOICE

1. The most common cause of death in children outside the newborn period is:
   a. Sudden infant death syndrome (SIDS)
   b. Trauma and respiratory conditions
   c. Congenital heart disease
   d. Cancer
2. Most cardiopulmonary arrests in children result from failure of the:
   a. Urinary system
   b. Cardiovascular system
   c. Respiratory system
   d. Endocrine system
3. Magical thinking is primarily associated with which period of development?
   a. Infants (less than 1 year)
   b. Toddlers (15 months to 3 years)
   c. Small children (4 to 7 years)
   d. Adolescents
4. When examining adolescents, it is most important to:
   a. Respect their privacy and shyness.
   b. Relax them with casual conversation.
   c. Be assertive to avoid resistance to questions.
   d. Be upbeat and familiar with them.
5. When examining small children, it is advisable to:
   a. Ask the parents to leave the room.
   b. Hold them on your lap.
   c. Leave them on the parents' lap.
   d. Do it quickly to avoid problems.
6. In small children the focused (secondary) assessment should proceed:
   a. In the same manner as in an adult.
   b. In a toe-to-head survey.
   c. Briskly to avoid prolonged exposure.
   d. Very slowly to avoid agitation.
7. The narrowest part of the upper airway in infants is the:
   a. Epiglottis
   b. Trachea
   c. Thyroid cartilage
   d. Cricoid cartilage
8. To open the airway of the infant, place the head in the:
   a. Hyperflexed position
   b. Extended position
   c. Flexed position
   d. Sniffing or neutral position
9. Hyperextension of an infant's airway may result in:
   a. Kinking and obstruction
   b. Rupture of the larynx
   c. Dislocation of the cervical spine
   d. Increased intracranial pressure

10. Infants (up to 1 year) have an average respiratory rate of approximately:
    a. 12 to 20 breaths/min
    b. 20 to 25 breaths/min
    c. 25 to 30 breaths/min
    d. 30 to 40 breaths/min
11. Infants breathe predominantly through the:
    a. Nose
    b. Mouth
    c. Pursed lips
    d. Cheeks
12. During ventilation, you must be careful to observe:
    a. Pupillary response
    b. Skin color
    c. Capillary refilling time
    d. Chest rise
13. When ventilating an infant, care should be taken *not* to overventilate because infants are more subject to:
    a. Pneumothorax
    b. Gastric distention
    c. Hemothorax
    d. Pulmonary contusions
14. Nasal flaring and retractions are signs of:
    a. Increased work of breathing
    b. Difficulty with exhalation
    c. Chest wall injury
    d. Hyperventilation
15. High-concentration oxygen therapy for children older than 1 year:
    a. Is contraindicated.
    b. May cause blindness.
    c. Is appropriate if needed.
    d. Is never needed.
16. As a general rule, the width of a blood pressure cuff applied to an infant or child should cover approximately what fraction of the length of the upper arm?
    a. 1/4
    b. 1/3
    c. 2/3
    d. 1/2
17. The American College of Surgeons defines a systolic blood pressure less than _____ mm Hg with tachycardia and cool skin as an indicator of shock in children.
    a. 50
    b. 70
    c. 80
    d. 90

18. Infants and children have a baseline metabolic rate _____ than adults.
    a. higher
    b. lower
19. Because of their healthier compensatory mechanisms, children maintain their blood pressure until they lose almost:
    a. 20% of blood volume
    b. 30% of blood volume
    c. 40% of blood volume
    d. 50% of blood volume
20. A crowing, high-pitched sound made on inspiration that is suggestive of upper airway obstruction is called:
    a. Grunting
    b. Snoring
    c. Wheezing
    d. Stridor
21. A rhythmic sound heard at the end of exhalation that may be mistaken for whining is called:
    a. Grunting
    b. Snoring
    c. Wheezing
    d. Stridor
22. The inward depression of muscular areas and their attached ribs, which are drawn inward and reflect an increased work at breathing, is called:
    a. Thoracic paradox
    b. Myotonia
    c. Retractions
    d. Myopia
23. High-pitched "musical" sounds caused by narrowing of the lower airways obstructing airflow are called:
    a. Rales
    b. Stridor
    c. Wheezing
    d. Grunting
24. A viral infection affecting the larynx, trachea, and bronchi that can cause airway narrowing, especially at the level of the cricoid ring, is called:
    a. Bronchiolitis
    b. Pharyngitis
    c. Croup
    d. Epiglottitis
25. Croup is most common from ages:
    a. 6 months to 3 years
    b. Newborn to 4 years
    c. 1 year to 8 years
    d. Newborn to 11 years
26. Epiglottitis is an acute bacterial infection of the epiglottis that has a rapid onset of approximately:
    a. 2 to 4 hours
    b. 1 to 2 hours
    c. 10 to 12 hours
    d. 24 to 72 hours
27. Which of the following is *not* a common sign of acute epiglottitis?
    a. High fever
    b. Sore throat
    c. Difficulty in swallowing
    d. Absent breath sounds on one side
28. The child with epiglottitis is frequently sitting upright and leaning forward, resting the chin on the arms, called the:
    a. Fowler's position
    b. Recumbent position
    c. Semi-Fowler's position
    d. Tripod position
29. A major contraindication in the management of acute epiglottitis is:
    a. Administering high-concentration oxygen.
    b. Examining the pharynx with a tongue blade.
    c. Humidifying oxygen during administration.
    d. None of the above.
30. When faced with a child who has a complete airway obstruction from acute epiglottitis or croup, you should:
    a. Administer back blows and chest thrusts.
    b. Attempt ventilation with the bag-mask.
    c. Initiate rapid transport.
    d. Both b and c.
31. A child with a foreign body airway obstruction who is alert and demonstrating effective air exchange should be managed by:
    a. A deep finger sweep to the upper airway
    b. Back blows and chest thrusts
    c. Transport only
    d. Positive-pressure ventilation
32. The correct management of a complete foreign body airway obstruction in a conscious infant is:
    a. Back blows
    b. Chest thrusts
    c. Finger sweep
    d. Both a and b
33. The correct position for an infant while administering back blows is:
    a. Supporting the head in your hand.
    b. Resting on your arm and thigh.
    c. The head in the dependent position.
    d. All of the above.
34. Which of the following signs is (are) associated with a partial airway obstruction with poor air exchange?
    a. A weak, ineffective cough
    b. Stridor
    c. Cyanosis
    d. All of the above
35. The correct position for a chest thrust while treating an infant with a complete foreign body airway obstruction is:
    a. One fingerbreadth above the xiphoid
    b. One fingerbreadth below the nipple line
    c. The nipple line
    d. The upper half of the breastbone

150

36. When a conscious infant with a complete airway obstruction becomes unconscious, you should first:
    a. Attempt to ventilate, and observe for chest excursion.
    b. Perform a jaw lift, examine airway, and perform a finger sweep if you visualize a foreign body.
    c. Administer four back blows and four chest thrusts.
    d. Check for a brachial pulse to establish the need for cardiac compressions.
37. The primary disease(s) affecting the lower airways in pediatric patients is (are):
    a. Asthma
    b. Bronchiolitis
    c. Pneumonia
    d. All of the above
38. Asthmatic attacks in children can be triggered by:
    a. Upper respiratory infections
    b. Allergies
    c. Medication withdrawal
    d. All of the above
39. Asthmatic children with difficult breathing who become sleepy and lie down should receive:
    a. Positive-pressure ventilation
    b. Humidified oxygen
    c. Nebulized oxygen
    d. Oxygen by nasal catheter
40. Anatomically, foreign bodies that enter the lower airway are more likely to enter the:
    a. Right main stem bronchus
    b. Left main stem bronchus
41. As in the adult, the preferred method for opening the airway of an infant and child is the:
    a. Jaw thrust
    b. Head-tilt/chin-lift
    c. Head-tilt/neck-lift
    d. Chin pull
42. While performing the maneuver described in question 41, the head should be placed in the:
    a. Hyperextended position
    b. Extended position
    c. Sniffing or neutral position
    d. Slightly flexed position
43. When providing positive-pressure ventilation in an infant, you should breathe at a rate of 1 breath every:
    a. 4 to 6 seconds
    b. 3 to 5 seconds
    c. 2 to 4 seconds
    d. 1 to 2 seconds
44. While ventilating a patient with a bag-mask resuscitator, if you note air leakage through the pop-off valve, you should:
    a. Use your mouth.
    b. Tape the valve closed.
    c. Use a nonrebreather mask.
    d. Do nothing and continue ventilating.
45. When caring for a young drowning patient found in shallow water, you should automatically treat the child as if he had:
    a. Kidney damage
    b. Cervical spine injury
    c. Diabetes
    d. A bacterial infection
46. SIDS is often confused with:
    a. Choking
    b. Child abuse
    c. Drowning
    d. Overdose
47. A common cause of seizures in small children is:
    a. Overdose
    b. Fever
    c. Aspiration
    d. Vomiting
48. The most common internal organ injured in children is the:
    a. Heart
    b. Lungs
    c. Spleen
    d. Liver
49. The leading cause of death in children age 1 to 14 years is:
    a. SIDS
    b. Drowning
    c. Trauma
    d. Airway obstruction
50. End-organ perfusion of the brain is best evaluated through the:
    a. Level of consciousness
    b. Capillary refill
    c. Reflexes
    d. Pupils
51. Which of the following statements best describes the EMT's role in reporting child abuse?
    a. The EMT is legally responsible for reporting child abuse in every state.
    b. The EMT is not legally responsible for reporting child abuse in every state but has an ethical responsibility.
    c. The EMT has neither an ethical nor a legal responsibility for reporting child abuse.
    d. The EMT should limit activities to care of injuries and not attend to social problems.
52. Because caring for seriously injured children can result in psychological trauma to the health care provider, a useful method of prevention for you as EMT is to:
    a. Treat the clinical condition without focusing on the nature of the event.
    b. Involve yourself in activities that will help you forget the disturbing events.
    c. Seek participation in an organized debriefing process after exposure to serious childhood injuries.
    d. Focus on the positive aspects of your interventions rather than the nature of the injury or illness.

Chapter **25** **Infants and Children**

MATCHING

Questions 53-56. Match the appearance of a bruise in column A with the age of the bruise in column B.

Column A	Column B
53. _____ Yellow/brown	a. 1 to 3 days
54. _____ Red/blue	b. 3 to 7 days
55. _____ Brown to clearing	c. 7 days
56. _____ Purple	d. 3 weeks

SHORT ANSWER

Questions 57-64. List the eight possible signs of early respiratory distress.

57. _____

_____

58. _____

_____

59. _____

_____

60. _____

_____

61. _____

_____

62. _____

_____

63. _____

_____

64. _____

_____

Questions 65-68. List the four key signs of respiratory failure.

65. _____

_____

66. _____

_____

67. _____

_____

68. _____

_____

TRUE/FALSE

69. _____ Central cyanosis is a sign of low oxygen saturation of the hemoglobin in the blood.

70. _____ The SAMPLE history is not used in the evaluation of a child.

71. _____ Normal capillary refill (no more than 2 seconds) in a child is an indication of good perfusion.

72. _____ A very high fever in a child is the mechanism that may trigger a seizure.

73. _____ A child with a high fever should be cooled by covering the child with a cloth soaked with tepid water.

74. _____ A seizure caused by a toxic ingestion, such as from lead or nicotine, is an idiopathic seizure.

75. _____ If an infant sustains a significant head injury and requires airway management, the best method to open the airway is the head-tilt/chin-lift method.

76. _____ The most common internal injury in childhood is rupture of the spleen.

CASE SCENARIOS

Questions 77 to 79 are based on the following scenario.

You respond to a call and find an alert 2-year-old boy who appears to be in severe respiratory distress. On physical examination you note a barking cough, nasal flaring, intercostal retractions, and stridor. The mother tells you that he had a recent upper respiratory infection and woke up during the night with difficulty breathing.

77. Based on the history and signs and symptoms, you strongly suspect:
    a. Asthma
    b. Epiglottitis
    c. Croup
    d. Airway obstruction

78. The most important prehospital treatment of this patient is:
    a. Administering humidified oxygen.
    b. Administering positive-pressure ventilation.
    c. Suctioning the airway.
    d. Placing in the head-down position.

79. The most appropriate way to transport this patient is:
    a. Supine with the mother present.
    b. Supine; no parent should accompany the patient in the ambulance.
    c. Sitting on the mother's lap.
    d. Sitting on the stretcher, in a position of comfort, with the mother present.

Questions 80 and 81 are based on the following scenario.

A 6-year-old boy was struck by an automobile and thrown 10 feet. He is lying supine and is responsive to painful but not verbal stimuli. There is delayed capillary refill, and his skin is pale, cool, and sweaty. His vital signs are pulse 150 beats/min and thready, blood pressure 60/40 mm Hg, and respirations 34 breaths/min and shallow. There is no accessory muscle use or distended neck veins. Breath sounds are equal bilaterally.

80. Management of this child should include:
    a. Oxygen by nonrebreather mask
    b. Bag-mask ventilation
    c. Ventilation with a manually triggered resuscitator
    d. Humidified oxygen by face mask
81. Based on the vital signs, you would suspect blood loss of about:
    a. 10%
    b. 15%
    c. 20%
    d. 40%

Questions 82 and 83 are based on the following scenario.

You respond to a 5-month-old female infant in cardiopulmonary arrest with mottling of the skin in the dependent areas of the body. The parents state they put her to bed an hour ago and found her like this when they checked on her 10 minutes before your arrival. They say the infant recently had an upper respiratory infection.

82. This infant's condition has most likely been caused by:
    a. Abuse
    b. Choking
    c. SIDS
    d. Heart failure
83. Your action should be to:
    a. Wait for the police to arrive because the child is irreversibly dead.
    b. Perform cardiopulmonary resuscitation and transport the baby to the hospital.
    c. Not touch or move the infant to preserve evidence.
    d. Record the parents' statements carefully and give them to the police on arrival.

Questions 84 to 86 are based on the following scenario.

You respond to a 3-year-old girl with high fever, a sore throat, difficulty swallowing, and inspiratory stridor. She is sitting upright and leaning forward with her weight distributed on her hands, her mouth open, her tongue protruding, and her chin thrust forward. She is restless and drooling and has a flushed face. Her breath sounds are diminished, but no wheezes or rhonchi are present.

84. Based on the patient history and signs/symptoms, you strongly suspect:
    a. Bronchiolitis
    b. Epiglottitis
    c. Croup
    d. Asthma

85. The most important immediate action is to:
    a. Administer humidified oxygen.
    b. Examine the lower airway.
    c. Suction the lower airway.
    d. Place her in the supine position.
86. If this patient were to become completely obstructed, you would:
    a. Perform abdominal thrusts.
    b. Attempt forced ventilations.
    c. Perform a finger sweep.
    d. Perform back blows.

Questions 87 to 90 are based on the following scenario.

You respond to an 11-month-old girl who developed acute respiratory distress while playing with her toys in her crib. She appears to be crying, but no sounds are emitted from her airway. The parents tell you she has had no illness up to this event. Your physical examination reveals chest movements without air exchange at the mouth and nose. Her lips are cyanotic, but there are no other obvious physical signs.

87. Based on the patient history and signs/symptoms, you strongly suspect:
    a. Foreign body obstruction
    b. Anaphylaxis
    c. Bronchiolitis
    d. Sleep apnea
88. The most important immediate action is to:
    a. Administer humidified oxygen.
    b. Examine the lower airway.
    c. Suction the lower airway.
    d. Administer up to 5 back blows and 5 chest thrusts.
89. You continue your efforts without success, and the child becomes unconscious. You should first:
    a. Examine the airway.
    b. Administer positive-pressure ventilation.
    c. Perform chest thrusts.
    d. Perform back blows.
90. Two minutes later you are able to ventilate the patient effectively, but you note that there is no pulse. When beginning compressions, you should position your fingers:
    a. One fingerbreadth above the nipple line
    b. One fingerbreadth below the nipple line
    c. Directly at the nipple line
    d. Just above the xiphoid process

Chapter **25** **Infants and Children**

26 Ambulance Operations

MULTIPLE CHOICE

1. The superior braking technique when driving an ambulance is:
   a. Left foot braking
   b. Right foot braking
   c. Dominant foot braking
   d. Alternate foot braking
2. Palming the wheel in a turn represents a:
   a. Poor driving habit
   b. Method of stable turning
   c. Method for "feeling" the turn
   d. Crash avoidance technique
3. Exemptions of traffic regulations provided by law for persons driving emergency vehicles are best described as:
   a. Necessary evils
   b. Privileges
   c. Protections from crashes
   d. Legal protections
4. The correct position of a lap belt is across the:
   a. Umbilicus
   b. Thigh
   c. Pelvic girdle
   d. Upper thigh
5. The chances of being seriously injured by a seat belt are approximately 1 in _____ crashes.
   a. 5
   b. 10
   c. 50
   d. 200
6. Emergency lights and sirens:
   a. Are necessary to relieve the operator of liability in case of an incident.
   b. Are most effective in low-light situations, such as at dawn or dusk.
   c. Do not relieve the operator of liability in the event of an incident.
   d. Are most effective at high speeds.
7. The most effective colors for rear-facing warning lamps are:
   a. Amber and blue
   b. Red and white
   c. Red and yellow
   d. Yellow and white
8. Four-way hazard lights:
   a. Should not be used in a moving vehicle.
   b. Should be turned off when the vehicle is parked.
   c. Are necessary in a moving ambulance.
   d. Are most effective in low-light situations.

9. The most effective warning lights are mounted:
   a. Just above the rear bumper
   b. On the roof
   c. At eye level to other drivers
   d. In the outermost corners of the vehicle
10. The sound pattern of a siren in a moving ambulance is best described as a:
    a. Circle with the siren at the center
    b. Square with the siren at the center
    c. Cone ahead of the vehicle
    d. Straight line in front of the vehicle
11. At 60 mph, the sound emitted from an ambulance siren:
    a. Moves more quickly through the air.
    b. Barely precedes the ambulance.
    c. Is louder on the sides of the vehicle.
    d. Will not be heard inside the ambulance.
12. The sweaty palms, rapid pulse, and tense muscles felt by the operator of an emergency vehicle when the siren is switched on can cause the operator immediately to begin speeding. This response is the result of:
    a. Endorphin release
    b. Adrenaline release
    c. Physical demands of driving
    d. Vagal stimulation
13. An escort vehicle should be used only when:
    a. The ambulance is traveling at high speeds.
    b. The operator is unfamiliar with the route.
    c. Police are available.
    d. There is more than one ambulance.
14. The two major control tasks of an emergency vehicle operator are speed control and:
    a. Vehicle balance
    b. Braking
    c. Radio communications
    d. Directional control
15. Van ambulances with raised tops:
    a. Have decreased wind resistance.
    b. Have a higher center of gravity.
    c. Are more stable during turns.
    d. Usually have steel roof skins.
16. When suddenly braking an ambulance, the rear brakes:
    a. Are considerably less effective than the front.
    b. Do most of the braking.
    c. Brake equally with the front brakes.
    d. Allow for better directional control.
17. When the brakes lock, the wheels stop turning and:
    a. Centrifugal force is lost.
    b. The stopping distance is decreased.
    c. Stopping friction is reduced.
    d. Momentum is lost.

155

18. A good way to judge the correct traveling distance between your ambulance and the vehicle in front of you in dry weather is to observe the vehicle as it passes a fixed object (e.g., telephone pole) and then be able to count _____ seconds before you reach the same object.
    a. 2
    b. 4
    c. 10
    d. 12
19. On icy roads, the rule in question 18 is increased to:
    a. 6 seconds
    b. 12 seconds
    c. 20 seconds
    d. 30 seconds
20. Most emergency vehicle crashes occur:
    a. On highways
    b. At the scene of the crash
    c. En route to a crash
    d. At intersections
21. If sterile supplies such as bandages or dressings become wet, they should be:
    a. Dried in an autoclave.
    b. Air-dried.
    c. Discarded.
    d. Dried under ultraviolet light.
22. The precautions taken to prevent spread of infectious disease are called:
    a. Infection control
    b. Infectious protection
    c. Infection guarding
    d. Infection barriers
23. The first phase of an ambulance call is:
    a. Documentation
    b. Dispatch
    c. Preparation
    d. Response

MATCHING

Match the ambulance type in column A with the descriptions in column B.

Column A	Column B
24. _____ Type I	a. Van-type ambulance.
25. _____ Type II	b. Modular patient compartment with van chassis.
26. _____ Type III	c. Modular patient compartment with truck chassis.

FILL IN THE BLANK

27. One hour from the time of injury to arrival at definitive care is called the _____ _____.
28. When approaching a medivac helicopter, you should always approach from the _____.

CASE SCENARIOS

Questions 29 to 31 refer to the following scenario.
You respond to a call for a farm incident in a rural area of your county. You encounter a 32-year-old man who was operating a plow in the field when the plow rolled over, pinning the patient under the machinery by his left leg. Although you cannot readily extricate the patient, you observe that his arm is severely mangled, and you cannot feel any distal pulses. The nearest trauma center is 90 minutes away by ground ambulance, and you anticipate a 30- to 60-minute extrication process.

29. Use of a helicopter for rapid transport is:
    a. Not indicated because the patient will not be extricated within the "platinum 10 minutes."
    b. Not indicated because the patient will not arrive at a trauma center within the "golden hour."
    c. Not indicated because the drive time to the hospital is less than 2 hours.
    d. Indicated because of the patient's injury combined with the extended transport time.
30. Once the patient is extricated from the machinery, you learn that the helicopter has an estimated arrival time of 5 minutes. You should:
    a. Defer any further care until the helicopter personnel arrive at the scene.
    b. Begin transport and cancel the helicopter.
    c. Initiate any treatment indicated, package the patient, and await the arrival of the helicopter.
    d. Prepare the landing zone by placing flares around the chosen landing area.
31. Once the helicopter arrives, you should *not* approach the helicopter unless:
    a. You can approach from the rear.
    b. You are directed to approach by the flight team and you maintain eye contact with the pilot.
    c. The helicopter is shut down and the rotors are secured by tie-down cords by the flight crew.
    d. Directed by the incident commander on the scene.

Questions 32 to 34 refer to the following scenario.
You respond to a call for an injured logger. As you respond to the rural scene, you round a curve in the road and see the scene blocked by a logging truck in the road. You apply the brakes immediately, and as you continue pressure on the brake pedal, you feel the pedal vibrating. Your vehicle is equipped with antilock brakes.

32. You should:
    a. Immediately take your foot off the brake to prevent an uncontrollable skid.
    b. Maintain pressure on the brake pedal because this sensation is normal when the antilock feature is engaged.
    c. Immediately pump the brake pedal to prevent an uncontrollable skid.
    d. Apply the emergency brake.

33. You arrive at the scene and observe that your patient is lying on his side approximately 30 yards off the road in the trees, approximately 20 feet below the level of the road. You should:
    a. Immediately summon a helicopter because this is the only way to extricate the patient.
    b. Safely make your way to the patient and evaluate his injuries.
    c. Wait with your ambulance until the high-angle rescue team can arrive.
    d. Place the patient on a scoop stretcher, and use a come-along attached to the vehicle's bumper to pull the patient up to the road.

34. The patient is safely and rapidly extricated and requires hospital care. The optimal time from injury to arrival at the operating room is sometimes referred to as the:
    a. Prime time
    b. Critical minutes
    c. Magic minutes
    d. Golden hour

27 Gaining Access

1. The term used to describe an extrication that can be accomplished with hand tools or skills such as opening locks is called:
   a. Disentanglement
   b. Simple or light extrication
   c. Strategic access
   d. Rapid extrication

2. Because of the possibility of spilled gasoline at a motor vehicle crash site, the *least* appropriate method of securing the scene is through the use of:
   a. Reflectors
   b. Flares
   c. Road cones
   d. Battery-operated lights

3. Blocks of wood used to stabilize vehicles are commonly called:
   a. Stacking blocks
   b. Cribbing
   c. Stabilizers
   d. Construction blocks

4. While attempting to gain further access through a vehicle window, the patient inside should be protected by:
   a. Moving the patient away from the window.
   b. Tilting the car away from the patient.
   c. Covering the patient with a rescue blanket.
   d. Shattering the window from the inside out.

5. On gaining access to the interior of a crash vehicle, you find a patient who is short of breath, pale, cool and sweaty, and hypotensive, with respiratory rate of 22 breaths/min. Your immediate reaction is to:
   a. Apply oxygen and a vest-type device.
   b. Rapidly extricate the patient.
   c. Apply the pneumatic antishock garment before extrication.
   d. Begin positive-pressure ventilation.

6. The simplest and best method for creating room between the driver and the steering wheel is to:
   a. Cut the steering wheel away.
   b. Slide the seat back.
   c. Distort the steering wheel.
   d. Cut the steering wheel post off.

7. One method of reducing the number of glass shards when breaking a car window is to:
   a. Wet the window.
   b. Tape the corners.
   c. Apply contact paper.
   d. Heat the window.

8. You respond to a call at a railroad yard and are told that two men have fallen inside a huge tanker. You climb to the top of the tanker and look down inside to see the two men approximately 15 feet below you. They do not respond when you call out to them. Your immediate action should be to:
   a. Enter the car with a nonrebreather mask on your face.
   b. Allow oxygen to flow through tubing into the tanker to clear the environment, then enter.
   c. Lower your partner with a rope to allow for rapid removal.
   d. Maintain a safe distance from the opening into the tanker, and contact a rescue unit with self-contained breathing apparatus equipment.

9. The purpose of extrication is to:
   a. Free a person who is entrapped in his or her surroundings.
   b. Preserve evidence at the scene.
   c. Provide fracture care away from the crash site.
   d. Allow for easier access to the airway.

10. When the EMT is working with rescue personnel at an incident requiring patient extrication, which of the following is true?
    a. Patient care precedes extrication unless delayed movement would endanger life.
    b. Extrication precedes patient care unless there are signs of uncontrolled bleeding.
    c. Careful packaging of the patient for removal is the responsibility of rescue personnel.
    d. EMTs should first attend to the patients who do not need extrication.

11. At the scene of a motor vehicle crash, in general the greatest threat to the personal safety of the EMT is:
    a. Cuts from broken glass
    b. Oncoming traffic
    c. Fire
    d. Toxic contamination

12. In general, assuming side access to a vehicle (through a door or open window) is *not* possible, what access point represents the next best alternative?
    a. Rear or front windshield
    b. Roof
    c. Floor
    d. Trunk

13. As you approach a car that was involved in a motor vehicle crash, your quick inspection that identifies if the patients are moving or conscious is called a(n):
    a. Windshield survey
    b. Initial (primary) assessment
    c. Detailed assessment
    d. Focused (secondary) assessment

CASE SCENARIOS

Questions 14 to 17 refer to the following scenario.
You respond to a call and find two cars in a head-on collision. You note that the passengers and driver of car #1 are ambulating and talking to bystanders. The passenger from car #2 appears in severe distress, and the driver appears to be dead.

14. The first action you should take when approaching the scene of a motor vehicle crash is to:
    a. Immediately call a tow truck for assistance.
    b. Call for additional units.
    c. Perform a windshield survey.
    d. Park your vehicle 500 feet from the scene.

15. In this crash situation, your first action on leaving the ambulance is to:
    a. Evaluate the passenger of car #2.
    b. Stabilize the cervical spine of the passenger from car #2.
    c. Make sure the scene is safe.
    d. Perform cardiopulmonary resuscitation on the driver of car #2.

16. On approaching car #2, you note that all the doors are jammed, the windows are closed, and the passenger is too confused to cooperate in opening the door. You should gain access to the patient by:
    a. Breaking the windshield.
    b. Cutting through the floor.
    c. Cutting through the roof.
    d. Breaking the rear driver-side window.

17. After you have gained access and pried open the door of car #2, you find the passenger in severe respiratory distress, with paradoxical breathing and pale, cool, and sweaty skin. Your immediate action should be to:
    a. Apply a pneumatic antishock garment.
    b. Apply a short spine board.
    c. Rapidly extricate the patient.
    d. Perform a secondary survey.

Questions 18 to 20 refer to the following scenario.
On arriving at the scene of a motor vehicle crash, you encounter a car with flames coming from beneath the hood. You note a driver and two passengers who are trapped in the car.

18. Your immediate action should be to:
    a. Attempt to extinguish the fire.
    b. Cut a flap in the door to gain access.
    c. Break the front windshield to gain access.
    d. Cut a roof flap to gain access.

19. By the time your patients are in the ambulance, you note that they are all exhibiting signs of respiratory distress. You suspect:
    a. Cyanide poisoning
    b. First-degree burns
    c. Carbon monoxide poisoning
    d. Hyperthermia

20. The most important treatment for these patients is:
    a. Humidified oxygen by a mask
    b. Oxygen by a nonrebreather mask
    c. Nasal cannula oxygen
    d. Cool compresses to their face

Questions 21 and 22 refer to the following scenario.
You respond to a crash scene and find a small, late-model sport utility vehicle (SUV) back on its wheels after rolling over at least once. There is only one vehicle involved. The SUV's driver is sitting behind the steering wheel and seems dazed. The scene appears to be safe. You are able to gain access to the vehicle easily through the driver's side door. The patient is wearing a lap/shoulder belt, and the airbags have not deployed.

21. The safest way to approach the patient and provide safety from the airbag is to:
    a. Trigger the airbag before entering the vehicle.
    b. Have the fire department cut the battery cables, which will ensure that the airbags cannot deploy.
    c. If available, place a protective cover over the steering wheel airbag, and maintain a safe distance from the steering wheel.
    d. There is no need for concern; the airbag cannot deploy if the vehicle is stopped.

22. You have provided rescuer and patient safety and begin your patient evaluation. Your patient complains of head and neck pain. His vital signs are pulse 82 beats/min and regular, blood pressure 136/78 mm Hg, and respiratory rate 16 breaths/min, full and regular. The best way to remove this patient from the SUV is:
    a. Move the patient directly onto a long spine board.
    b. Immobilize the patient in a vest-type device, then remove him to a long spine board.
    c. Allow the patient to step out of the car and sit on your stretcher.
    d. Perform a rapid extrication.

28 Disasters and Hazardous Materials

MULTIPLE CHOICE

1. The primary responsibility of an EMT at a hazardous materials incident is:
   a. Containment
   b. Decontamination
   c. Emergency medical care
   d. Removal

2. You smell a strange odor when approaching a scene involving a transportation vehicle; you should first:
   a. Relocate upwind and assess the scene from a distance.
   b. Apply your self-contained breathing apparatus gear and approach the scene to perform an assessment.
   c. Approach the scene and assess.
   d. Contact Chemtec immediately to have an expert come to the scene.

3. When reacting to a documented HAZMAT incident, it is important to establish a patient treatment and transport location called a:
   a. Command center
   b. Staging area
   c. Communications area
   d. Triage area

4. The bill of lading is most often found:
   a. In the cab of the vehicle or with the driver
   b. Posted on the back end of the vehicle
   c. Posted on the side of the vehicle
   d. Posted on the front of the vehicle

5. To minimize damage to the environment, the EMT may assist rescue personnel to prevent runoff by use of:
   a. A dike or trench
   b. Irrigation into the sewer
   c. An ABC fire extinguisher to neutralize the runoff
   d. Vacuum devices

6. Which of the following best represents a closed disaster?
   a. Plane crash on a mountain with no access road
   b. Building collapse in a city
   c. Burning building
   d. Multiple-car collision on a highway

7. A predetermined response system with neighboring communities that ensures a large-scale response of emergency vehicles during a disaster best describes a:
   a. Transfer agreement
   b. Mutual aid agreement
   c. Cross-coverage plan
   d. Mass casualty incident strategy

8. The sorting of casualties of war or other disaster to determine the priority of need and proper place of treatment best defines:
   a. Categorization
   b. Stacking
   c. Triage
   d. Designation

9. The secondary triage area is where treatment occurs and where:
   a. Patients are staged for transport.
   b. Dead patients are identified.
   c. The command post is ideally located.
   d. The communications center is established.

10. When a disaster victim fears death, perceives limited escape, and has no information about what happened, the likely outcome is:
    a. Suicide
    b. Depression
    c. Panic
    d. Psychosis

11. At the site of a disaster, drivers of emergency vehicles should:
    a. Participate in early triage and treatment.
    b. Park as close to the scene as possible.
    c. Remain with their vehicles.
    d. Report to the triage officer.

12. The rapid response of onlookers, rescuers, and press at the scene of a disaster that results in the blockage of traffic routes is called:
    a. Accident crowding
    b. Convergence
    c. Focal obstruction
    d. Central merge

13. The process of demobilizing response vehicles and apparatus for the purposes of returning them to normal community service is called:
    a. Recovery
    b. Remobilization
    c. Reintroduction
    d. Rehabilitation

14. The rebuilding of the community in a physical and emotional sense after a disaster, a process that includes critical incident stress debriefing, is referred to as:
    a. Reconstruction
    b. Rehabilitation
    c. Recovery
    d. Restoration

15. The three essential components of emergency services in disaster management are:
    a. Command, triage, and transport
    b. Triage, patient care, and transport
    c. Triage, communications, and patient care
    d. Command, control, and triage
16. The log that records the patient distribution to ambulances and hospital destination is called the:
    a. Major event log
    b. Logistics sheet
    c. Transportation log
    d. Destination log
17. At a disaster scene, the person whose function is to control traffic flow, gather supplies, stage additional vehicles, and communicate ambulance availability to the command post is the:
    a. Supply officer
    b. Transport officer
    c. Communication officer
    d. Triage officer
18. The process by which participants are allowed to express their feelings about the incident and thereby relieve the associated stress is called the:
    a. Catharsis
    b. Debriefing
    c. Critique
    d. Field exercise

MATCHING

Questions 19-22. Match the appropriate color triage tag in column A with the condition in column B.

Column A	Column B
19. _____ Red	a. Unconscious patient with head injury
20. _____ Yellow	b. Cardiac arrest patient
21. _____ Green	c. Multiple pelvic fractures
22. _____ Black	d. Fractured humerus

Questions 23-26. Match the type of training in column A to the expected role that an individual would play at the scene of a hazardous materials incident in column B.

Column A	Column B
23. _____ First responder/ awareness	a. Individual who would attempt to stop the release of a hazardous substance.
24. _____ Hazardous materials technician	b. Individual with highest level of training who has specific or direct knowledge of substances being released.
25. _____ Hazardous materials specialist	c. Individual who would respond to hazmat incident and is trained to contain the release from a safe distance.
26. _____ First responder/ operations	d. Individual likely to witness or discover a hazmat incident and then initiate an emergency response.

TRUE/FALSE

27. _____ A Level D suit provides for the highest level of respiratory protection when dealing with potential chemical contamination.
28. _____ Placards, which are affixed to the outside of the transport vehicle, identify the specific type of decontamination procedure to be followed if a patient becomes contaminated by the substance during shipping.
29. _____ Control zones are geographic areas at a hazardous materials incident that are based on safety and the degree of hazard.
30. _____ The principal patient management technique in the hot zone is patient decontamination.
31. _____ Once decontaminated, patients can be brought to the cold zone.
32. _____ The principal patient management technique in the warm zone is patient removal.
33. _____ Patients exposed to cyanide or organophosphates may require an immediate antidote.

CASE SCENARIOS

Questions 34 to 39 refer to the following scenario.
You and your partner are the first to arrive at the scene of a major airplane crash in a hilly, wooded area. At least 100 people were on the aircraft at the time of impact. The left wing of the plane is smoking. It is late fall at twilight and starting to snow lightly, and the wind is blowing strong from the north. The nearest hospital is about 20 minutes away, but there is only a single narrow road to access the area, and several cars belonging to

local residents are already beginning to block the road. Your partner is the driver.

34. This disaster can be described as:
    a. Open, active
    b. Closed, active
    c. Open, contained
    d. Closed, contained

35. As you and your partner arrive at the disaster scene:
    a. You should secure your vehicle, making sure that the road is not obstructed, and then you and your partner should begin to do a scene survey.
    b. Radio for additional assistance, then both stay in the ambulance until at least one other vehicle arrives.
    c. Both should drive back down the road to block further traffic and radio for assistance.
    d. Radio for police, fire, and rescue assistance, then both stay with the vehicle until firefighters arrive.

36. As the first arriving EMT, you or your partner will temporarily become the _____ officer.
    a. Command
    b. Triage
    c. Traffic
    d. Post

37. The best place for a temporary command post at this time would be:
    a. Near the right wing of the plane
    b. 200 yards south of the plane
    c. 200 yards north of the plane
    d. In a building half a mile away

38. Your partner discovers four injured patients: a 50-year-old unconscious man with a head injury, a 16-year-old boy in cardiac arrest, a 60-year-old man with bilateral fractures of the radius and ulna, and a 35-year-old man with an open fracture of the femur. Which patient should receive priority?
    a. 50-year-old man
    b. 16-year-old boy
    c. 35-year-old man
    d. 60-year-old man

39. The 16-year-old patient would be considered a _____ triage category.
    a. Red
    b. Yellow
    c. Green
    d. Black

Questions 40 to 44 refer to the following scenario.
You respond to a city street where a hot dog vendor's propane tank has exploded, causing more than 10 injuries. The truck is engulfed in flames. The scene is chaotic, with people running in every direction and screaming for help.

40. This disaster can be described as:
    a. Open, active
    b. Closed, active
    c. Open, contained
    d. Closed, contained

41. As you approach the disaster area, your first concern should be:
    a. Triaging and identifying the severely injured patients.
    b. Calling for additional assistance.
    c. Protecting yourself and bystanders.
    d. Staying with your vehicle until firefighters arrive.

42. Based on the conditions described, which service is likely to assume command?
    a. Emergency medical services
    b. Fire
    c. Police
    d. Other agency

43. You discover four injured patients: a 25-year-old man with 40% second- and third-degree burns, an unconscious 42-year-old man with an open chest wound, an 18-year-old woman in cardiac arrest, and a 58-year-old woman with a fracture of the radius. Rank these patients in order of priority treatment:
    1. 25-year-old man
    2. 42-year-old man
    3. 18-year-old woman
    4. 58-year-old woman
       a. 1, 3, 2, 4
       b. 2, 1, 4, 3
       c. 2, 3, 1, 4
       d. 1, 2, 3, 4

44. The 18-year-old patient would be considered a _____ triage category.
    a. Red
    b. Yellow
    c. Green
    d. Black

CROSSWORD PUZZLE

Puzzle 28-1

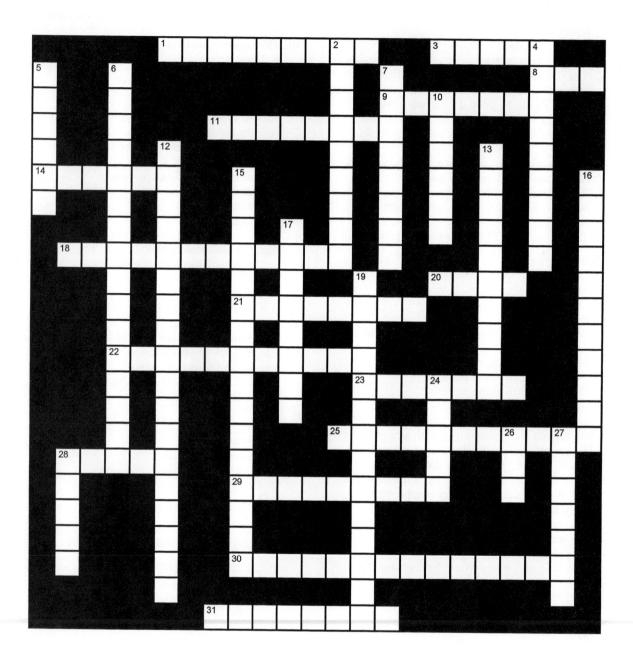

Across

1. Level of training appropriate for first responders likely to witness or discover a hazardous incident
3. Technique for quick primary triage
8. Disaster tag color for critical patients
9. Area in which contamination occurs
11. Area immediately surrounding the hot zone where decontamination occurs
14. Fully encapsulated, gas-tight body suit and SCBA are required in this classification of chemical protective clothing.
18. The weight of a volume of gas compared with an equal volume of air
20. National Fire Protection Association
21. Diamond-shaped signs that identify the classification of hazardous materials
22. Rebuilding of the community, both physically and emotionally
23. Sector where ambulances receive assignments of patients and hospital destination
25. Rapid gathering of onlookers, rescuers, and the press at the scene of a disaster
28. Boiling liquid-expanding vapor explosion
29. Entering the body by swallowing
30. Sector where physical and psychological care is rendered to rescuers
31. Area where staging of supplies and the command center is established

Down

2. Information is gathered in the rapid trauma survey during _____ triage.
4. Sector where major field medical aid is administered
5. Sector designed to deliver the equipment resources to the disaster scene
6. Drill in which participants try to solve problems in a roundtable forum
7. A 24 hr/day, 7 days/week resource for hazardous material information
10. To sort casualties in order of priority
12. Substances capable of creating harm
13. Entering the body through the skin
15. Ambulance staging and dispatch are this person's primary function.
16. The EMT's primary duty at a hazardous material incident
17. Sudden, catastrophic event producing great damage, loss, and distress
19. Sector responsible for overall activities related to moving patients and resources
24. Disaster tag color generally used for ambulatory patients
26. Environmental Protection Agency
27. The person ultimately in charge of the disaster response
28. Disaster tag color for patients in cardiac arrest

Chapter **28** **Disasters and Hazardous Materials**

29 Advanced Airway Management

MULTIPLE CHOICE

1. Which of the following does *not* constitute a function of the upper airway?
   a. Filtration
   b. Gas exchange
   c. Warming or cooling
   d. Humidification

2. The first bifurcation of the trachea produces the:
   a. Two bronchi, equal in length and angulation
   b. Four lobar bronchi
   c. Two bronchi, of which the left is longer and has a more acute angle than the right
   d. Two bronchi, of which the right is longer and has a more acute angle than the left

3. The primary respiratory center is located in the:
   a. Medulla
   b. Cerebral cortex
   c. Apneustic center
   d. Pneumotaxic center

4. When using a curved laryngoscope blade, it is inserted in the:
   a. Glottic opening
   b. Vallecula
   c. Carina
   d. Uvula

5. When visualizing the vocal cords, the best position for the head is:
   a. Over the end of the bed
   b. In a neutral position
   c. Flexed forward, chin to chest
   d. In the sniffing position

6. When advancing an endotracheal tube, it should be inserted:
   a. Until 1 inch is extended from the mouth
   b. Just until the cuff is past the vocal cords
   c. Until it cannot be advanced any farther
   d. Until 3 inches is extended from the mouth

7. After intubation the chest is being auscultated, and breath sounds are *not* being heard on one side. You should:
   a. Move the tube slightly ahead and reevaluate.
   b. Rotate the tube and reevaluate.
   c. Remove the tube completely.
   d. Move the tube back slightly and reevaluate.

8. In most cases, when the tube is inserted too far, it will lodge in the:
   a. Left bronchus
   b. Right bronchus
   c. Terminal bronchioles
   d. Carina

9. The respiratory structure that is palpable just above the sternum is the:
   a. Bronchus
   b. Trachea
   c. Carina
   d. Bronchiole

10. The structure that covers the trachea during swallowing to prevent aspiration is called the:
    a. Pharynx
    b. Epiglottis
    c. Thyroid cartilage
    d. Cricoid cartilage

11. The narrowest part of the upper airway in infants is the:
    a. Epiglottis
    b. Trachea
    c. Thyroid cartilage
    d. Cricoid cartilage

12. To open the airway of the infant, place the head in the:
    a. Hyperflexed position
    b. Extended position
    c. Flexed position
    d. Sniffing or neutral position

13. Hyperextension of an infant's airway may result in:
    a. Kinking and obstruction
    b. Rupture of the larynx
    c. Dislocation of the cervical spine
    d. Increased intracranial pressure

14. Infants breathe predominantly through the:
    a. Nose
    b. Mouth
    c. Pursed lips
    d. Cheeks

15. On inserting an oropharyngeal airway, the patient begins to gag and choke. Your next action should be to:
    a. Remove the airway.
    b. Use a smaller airway.
    c. Lubricate the airway.
    d. Tape the airway in place.

16. To ensure proper sizing, an oropharyngeal airway is measured from the center of the patient's mouth to the:
    a. Angle of the jaw
    b. Top of the ear
    c. Cheekbone
    d. Trachea

17. The endotracheal tubes for infants and small children are:
    a. More rigid
    b. More curved
    c. Differently shaped
    d. Uncuffed

18. When suctioning the upper airway, you should activate the negative pressure:
    a. When the tip is in the oropharynx
    b. Before insertion
    c. At the entrance of the mouth
    d. Halfway between the teeth and the pharynx
19. Lifting at the angles of the jaw while maintaining the head in the neutral inline position best describes the:
    a. Modified jaw thrust
    b. Head-tilt/chin-lift
    c. Chin pull
    d. Tongue-jaw lift
20. Tilting the head back with one hand while lifting the lower margin of the jaw with the index and middle fingers of the other hand best describes the:
    a. Jaw thrust without head tilt
    b. Chin-pull maneuver
    c. Head-tilt/neck-lift
    d. Head-tilt/chin-lift
21. The best way to remove liquid secretions from the airway in the field is by:
    a. Finger sweeps
    b. Back blows
    c. Portable suction
    d. Abdominal thrusts
22. When using a jaw thrust in conjunction with a bag-mask device, you can lift the mandible at the:
    a. Center of the chin
    b. Angle of the jaw
    c. Lower portion of the cheekbones
    d. Soft tissues of the mandible
23. To ensure proper sizing, a nasopharyngeal airway is measured from the nares to the:
    a. Angle of the jaw
    b. Top of the ear
    c. Cheekbone
    d. Larynx
24. The most common cause of airway obstruction in an unconscious patient is:
    a. A foreign body
    b. Anaphylaxis
    c. The tongue
    d. Aspiration
25. Airway obstruction caused by anaphylaxis is best managed by:
    a. Positive-pressure ventilation
    b. Back blows
    c. Chest thrusts
    d. Abdominal thrusts
26. The primary use of a nasogastric tube in the field is:
    a. When you are unable to ventilate an infant or child because of gastric distention.
    b. To clear the stomach of poisons.
    c. To remove liquids from the stomach to avoid aspiration.
    d. To prevent gastric insufflation while ventilating an infant.

27. The Sellick maneuver is performed by applying pressure to the:
    a. Trachea
    b. Cricoid ring
    c. Thyroid cartilage
    d. Epiglottis
28. The primary indication for orotracheal intubation in the field is:
    a. Protecting the airway of an unconscious patient.
    b. Routine prevention of aspiration of gastric contents.
    c. Suctioning the lower airway of a patient.
    d. Securing the airway and ventilating a patient in respiratory arrest.
29. Equipment used during orotracheal intubation to maintain the shape of the tube to aid placement of the tip into the glottic opening is called the:
    a. Pilot balloon
    b. Stylet
    c. Tube cylinder
    d. Murphy's eye
30. When using a straight laryngoscope blade, it is inserted beneath the:
    a. Glottic opening
    b. Vallecula
    c. Carina
    d. Epiglottis
31. A device used to confirm placement of an endotracheal tube by monitoring gases is called a(n):
    a. Pulse oximeter
    b. Blood gas monitor
    c. End-tidal carbon dioxide detector
    d. Ventilator monitor
32. Which of the following endotracheal tubes is appropriate for an average adult male?
    a. 5.0 mm
    b. 6.0 mm
    c. 8.0 mm
    d. 11.0 mm
33. Which of the following methods is used to size an endotracheal tube for a child?
    a. (16 plus child's age) divided by 4
    b. (12 plus child's age) divided by 2
    c. (10 plus child's age) divided by 3
    d. (8 plus child's age) divided by 4
34. A simple alternate method for sizing an endotracheal tube for an infant or child is:
    a. Comparing tube's diameter to child's little finger.
    b. Comparing tube's diameter to child's mouth opening.
    c. Comparing tube's length to child's index finger.
    d. Comparing tube's length to child's middle finger.
35. You should continually monitor heart rate during an intubation of an infant or child with a pulse because stimulation of the airway may cause:
    a. Bleeding and shock
    b. Ventricular fibrillation
    c. Slowing of the heart rate
    d. Rapid heart rhythms

168

36. Failure to note an esophageal intubation is most likely to result in:
   a. Aspiration
   b. Hypoxia and death
   c. Esophageal rupture
   d. Tear of the stomach
37. When securing the endotracheal tube, an oropharyngeal airway can be used to prevent:
   a. Occluding the tube if the patient bites down.
   b. Displacing the tongue into the airway.
   c. Dislodging the endotracheal tube.
   d. Injuring the teeth and gums.
38. The esophageal-tracheal Combitube (ETC):
   a. Is designed for use in patients older than 5 years.
   b. Is in the trachea after normal insertion.
   c. Requires the use of the laryngoscope for proper placement.
   d. Is inserted blindly.
39. The most significant complication when using the ETC is:
   a. Ventilation through the incorrect port after inserting the device
   b. Rupture of the trachea
   c. Trauma to the vocal cords
   d. Chipping or breaking of teeth
40. When inflating the cuffs on the ETC, you should use approximately:
   a. 10 to 20 mL in each cuff
   b. 10 to 20 mL in proximal cuff and 80 to 100 mL in distal cuff
   c. 80 to 100 mL in proximal cuff and 10 to 20 mL in distal cuff
   d. 80 to 100 mL in each cuff
41. When done properly, the laryngeal mask airway is inserted:
   a. With tip of the mask resting on upper end of the esophagus and surrounding opening of the larynx.
   b. In the trachea just below the vocal cords.
   c. In the esophagus.
   d. To maintain an airtight seal over the mouth and nose.
42. The laryngeal mask airway is indicated:
   a. For patients with a respiratory rate of more than 36 breaths/min.
   b. For patients without intravenous access who need rapid administration of medications through the airway.
   c. For patients who are apneic and unresponsive and do not have a cough or gag reflex.
   d. After the patient is successfully orally intubated with an endotracheal tube.
43. Which laryngoscope blade will be more helpful when intubating a 6-month-old child?
   a. Size 1 curved blade
   b. Size 1 straight blade
   c. Size 3 curved blade
   d. Size 3 straight blade

44. You have successfully intubated a 3-year-old child. You should:
   a. Secure the tube in place with a commercial holder; the tube does not have a cuff.
   b. Inflate the cuff with approximately 10 mL of air.
   c. Immediately insert an oral airway because the tongue is proportionally smaller in the child than in the adult.
   d. Ventilate with the appropriate-sized bag-mask device at least six times before auscultating breath sounds.

MATCHING

Questions 45-51. Match the term in column A with the correct description in column B.

Column A	Column B
45. _____ Vocal cords	a. Space between vocal cords
46. _____ Thyroid cartilage	b. Structure that creates voice
47. _____ Glottis	c. Commonly called "Adam's apple"
48. _____ Cricothyroid membrane	d. Disease when alveoli are damaged or destroyed
49. _____ Trachea	e. Structure that permits movement of food to the stomach
50. _____ Esophagus	f. Lies between the cricoid and thyroid cartilage
51. _____ Emphysema	g. Structure that permits movement of air from the larynx to the bronchi

Questions 52-57. Identify whether the assessment method in column A for endotracheal tube placement is a primary or secondary means of confirmation (column B).

Column A	Column B
52. _____ Direct visualization of tube passing between vocal cords.	a. Primary confirmation
53. _____ Carbon dioxide detectors.	b. Secondary confirmation
54. _____ Pulse oximetry.	
55. _____ Auscultation of breath sounds.	
56. _____ Observation of rise and fall of chest with ventilations.	
57. _____ Esophageal detector devices.	

Chapter **29** **Advanced Airway Management**

FILL IN THE BLANK

58. Voice is created by movement of air past the

    _____ _____.

59. Diffusion of gases occurs between the lungs and the circulatory system in the lungs in the structures

    called _____.

60. The effectiveness of ventilations is largely measured

    by _____ _____ levels in the blood.

61. The passage extending from the back of the nasal cavity down to the esophagus and larynx is called

    the _____.

62. The _____ _____ is used during positive-pressure ventilation to minimize gastric inflation and regurgitation.

SHORT ANSWER

Questions 63-66. List four complications of orotracheal intubation other than esophageal intubation.

63. _____

    _____

64. _____

    _____

65. _____

    _____

66. _____

    _____

TRUE/FALSE

67. _____ The cuff of an endotracheal tube should generally be filled with approximately 50 mL of air.

68. _____ The small hole at the end of the endotracheal tube is called Murphy's eye.

69. _____ The small hole at the end of the endotracheal tube is used to assist in securing the tube in place.

70. _____ In general, commercial devices are more likely to secure the tube in place than tape.

71. _____ A towel may be used to elevate the back of the head in infants and small children to facilitate placing the patient in the sniffing position.

72. _____ The pulse oximeter may give an inaccurate reading for a patient who has carbon monoxide poisoning.

73. _____ The esophageal-tracheal Combitube is indicated for apneic patients who are unresponsive and do not have a cough or gag reflex.

74. _____ For children younger than 8 years, an uncuffed endotracheal tube should be used.

CASE SCENARIOS

Questions 75 to 79 refer to the following scenario.
You arrive at the scene of a 4-year-old boy who was pulled from a swimming pool earlier. The patient was found at the bottom of the pool and was removed by his babysitter. The child had been swimming and did not dive into the pool. The police on scene are performing cardiopulmonary resuscitation.

75. The best way to provide ventilation to this patient is:
    a. Open the airway with a head-tilt/chin-lift and ventilate with a pocket mask without supplemental oxygen.
    b. Open the airway with a head-tilt/chin-lift and ventilate with a bag-mask device connected to 15 L/min oxygen.
    c. Open the airway with a jaw thrust and ventilate with a pocket mask without supplemental oxygen.
    d. Open the airway with a jaw thrust and ventilate with a bag-mask device connected to 15 L/min oxygen.

76. The best way to determine that positive-pressure ventilation is achieving your goal of good ventilation is to:
    a. Observe for a change in skin color from blue to pink.
    b. Connect this patient to a pulse oximeter.
    c. Watch for adequate chest rise.
    d. Perform a finger sweep.

77. Despite repeated attempts at positioning the patient, you continue to have difficulty adequately ventilating him. You decide to intubate the patient orally and select an endotracheal tube of size:
    a. 4.0
    b. 5.0
    c. 6.0
    d. 7.0

78. This endotracheal tube should:
    a. Not have a cuff, and a stylet must not be used.
    b. Not have a cuff, and a stylet can be used.
    c. Have a cuff, and a stylet must not be used.
    d. Have a cuff, and a stylet can be used.

79. After passing the endotracheal tube, you use an esophageal detector device to confirm tube placement. You should:
    a. Connect the device to the tube, compress the bulb, and if the bulb expands, the tube is probably correctly placed in the trachea.
    b. Connect the device to the tube, compress the bulb, and if the bulb expands, the tube is probably *incorrectly* placed in the esophagus.
    c. Compress the bulb, then connect the device to the tube, and if the bulb expands, the tube is probably correctly placed in the trachea.
    d. Compress the bulb, then connect the device to the tube, and if the bulb expands, the tube is probably *incorrectly* placed in the esophagus.

Questions 80 to 83 refer to the following scenario.
You respond to a call for a 53-year-old man who is unconscious at a ball field. His friends tell you that he suddenly clutched his chest and then became unconscious. You immediately evaluate the patient and determine that he is in cardiac arrest. You have your automated external defibrillator (AED) and basic/advanced airway equipment at the patient's side.

80. You should immediately:
    a. Begin positive-pressure ventilations.
    b. Intubate the patient.
    c. Connect the AED to the patient.
    d. Begin transport.

81. At the appropriate time during the call, you begin to intubate the patient. You should use a:
    a. No. 2 straight blade with a 6.0-mm endotracheal tube
    b. No. 2 curved blade with an 8.0-mm endotracheal tube
    c. No. 4 straight blade with a 6.0-mm endotracheal tube
    d. No. 4 curved blade with an 8.0-mm endotracheal tube

82. Once you have intubated the patient, you auscultate breath sounds and note absent sounds on the left side of the chest, no sounds over the epigastrium, and good sounds on the right side of the chest. The endotracheal tube is:
    a. In the esophagus
    b. In the left main stem bronchus
    c. In the right main stem bronchus
    d. Properly placed

83. Based on the location of the endotracheal tube, you should:
    a. Remove the tube and reintubate the patient.
    b. Secure the tube where it is and ventilate the patient.
    c. Push the tube slightly farther into the patient.
    d. Pull the tube a short way out of the patient.

30 Weapons of Mass Destruction and the EMT

MULTIPLE CHOICE

1. Preparation for all disasters must:
   a. Begin at the local level in each community.
   b. Be established by national laws and regulations.
   c. Be developed by the national disaster medical service.
   d. Acknowledge that federal response teams will be the first responders.

2. Which type of incident causes the most immediate havoc and destruction?
   a. Chemical agent
   b. Biologic agent
   c. Viral agent
   d. Bacterial agent

3. The index cases in a nuclear, biologic, or chemical (NBC) event include:
   a. The most recent victim of the attack
   b. The youngest patients
   c. The patients who are exposed but do not show any effects of the exposure
   d. Victims with severe effects or among the early fatalities

4. You are at the scene and encounter a patient who had contact with a suspicious white powder. The powder is visible on the table. You should:
   a. Immediately transport the exposed person to the hospital.
   b. Remain in the room until the police arrive and determine if the powder contains anthrax.
   c. Leave the area, cover your mouth and nose with a mask, and keep bystanders away until specially trained personnel arrive.
   d. Administer an atropine injector to the exposed patient.

5. Smallpox is considered to be a biologic warfare agent that:
   a. Is readily available and may be used by terrorists.
   b. Is currently not considered a major threat because the population has been vaccinated against smallpox.
   c. Can be spread by coughing and sneezing from an infected patient.
   d. Can be prevented if the EMT wears gloves when treating all patients.

6. Viral hemorrhagic fevers include:
   a. Marburg and Ebola viruses
   b. Rocky Mountain spotted fever and shingles
   c. Tularemia and encephalitis
   d. Meningitis and pneumococcal pneumonia

7. Tularemia is usually acquired by:
   a. Contact with poisonous plants
   b. Contact with poisonous coral in the ocean
   c. Bites by deerflies or ticks
   d. Ingestion of contaminated food

8. If used as a weapon of mass destruction, tularemia most likely would be spread by terrorists through what means?
   a. Vectors such as insect bites
   b. Aerosol
   c. Distribution of contaminated powder in the mail or in public places
   d. Contaminated stockpiles of antibiotics

9. Botulism results in a:
   a. Classic feet upward, ascending paralysis
   b. Generalized paralysis that affects the entire body simultaneously
   c. Classic head downward, descending paralysis
   d. Generalized weakness in the lower extremities that slowly progresses to paralysis

10. At room temperature, nerve agents are a:
    a. Volatile gas
    b. Crystalline powder
    c. Liquid
    d. Solid putty material similar to clay

11. The major threat from contact with the vapors from sarin gas is:
    a. Absorption through the skin
    b. Contamination of the eyes
    c. Ingestion through contaminated food
    d. Inhalation of the gas

12. The first step in decontaminating a victim exposed to a nerve agent, whether in vapor or liquid form, is usually:
    a. Removing the patient's clothing.
    b. Quickly irrigating the patient while still clothed.
    c. Quickly irrigating the patient while neutralizing the liquid with baking soda.
    d. Quickly covering the patient with a sterile burn sheet.

13. The first organs in the body that will show the effects of exposure to cyanide gas are:
    a. Heart and kidneys
    b. Lungs and heart
    c. Heart and brain
    d. Brain and lungs

14. Rapid onset of hyperpnea followed by seizures, loss of respirations, and death within 6 to 8 minutes is a classic example of exposure to:
    a. Nerve agents
    b. Cyanide gas
    c. Phosgene gas
    d. Chlorine gas
15. You are a rescuer equipped with full protective equipment and encounter patients in the hot zone, where you should provide:
    a. Full patient decontamination
    b. A complete START triage
    c. Treatment with the MARK I kit for severe nerve agent poisoning
    d. A detailed physical assessment
16. The *least* common type of radioactive emissions is:
    a. Alpha particles
    b. Beta particles
    c. Gamma rays
    d. Neutrons
17. The irreversible cardiovascular effects of acute radiation syndrome are seen if the patient has been exposed to approximately:
    a. 100 rem
    b. 400 rem
    c. 1000 rem
    d. 3000 rem

MATCHING

Questions 18-21. Match the type of chemical agent in column A with the clinical presentation of the patient in column B.

Column A	Column B
18. _____ Nerve agents	a. Pulmonary edema and shortness of breath, first noticed with exertion.
19. _____ Cyanide agents	b. Small pupils, muscle twitching, and secretions associated with rapid loss of consciousness, convulsions, and respiratory arrest.
20. _____ Sulfur mustard	c. Loss of consciousness, convulsions, and respiratory arrest, in some cases preceded by irritation of nasal passages and eyes.
21. _____ Pulmonary agents	d. Redness or erythema of the skin that develops into progressively larger blisters.

Questions 22-24. Match the unit of measurement in column A with the description in column B.

Column A	Column B
22. _____ roentgen	a. Measurement of the amount of radiation absorbed by the body.
23. _____ rad	b. Measurement of a charge in the air caused by ionizing radiation.
24. _____ rem	c. Unit equal to the absorbed dose in rad multiplied by modifying factors, which allows for some comparison of the effects of different types of radiation.

Questions 25-28. Match the type of radiation in column A with the description in column B.

Column A	Column B
25. _____ Alpha particles	a. High-energy electromagnetic radiation similar to x-rays but more energetic.
26. _____ Beta particles	b. Uncharged particles found in the nucleus of an atom.
27. _____ Gamma rays	c. Least penetrating form of radiation that can be stopped by a sheet of paper.
28. _____ Neutrons	d. Radiation that travels no more than a few feet but can be stopped by the skin, causing burns similar to thermal burns.

FILL IN THE BLANK

29. A "red flag" for an intentional event may be defined as _____ _____ (all with) _____, _____ (and at) _____.

30. If available, the best material to use as a shield against radiation is an apron made of _____.

31. You are the first to respond and discover a possible nuclear incident. Your first priority is to establish a _____ _____.

32. The organized system of dealing with a mass casualty incident that identifies the role of all responders is referred to as the _____ _____ _____.

SHORT ANSWER

Questions 33-35. List the three primary roles of the EMT relating to a potential nuclear, biologic, or chemical (NBC) event.

33. _____

_____

34. _____

_____

35. _____

_____

Questions 36-38. List the three major factors used by rescuers to limit exposure to radiation.

36. _____

_____

37. _____

_____

38. _____

_____

Questions 39-41. List the three purposes of decontamination for a victim who was contaminated with a radioactive material.

39. _____

_____

40. _____

_____

41. _____

_____

TRUE/FALSE

42. _____ Biologic agents are not infectious.
43. _____ All biologic agents are contagious.
44. _____ Use of personal protective equipment is the same for potential biologic agents as for general patient care.
45. _____ The use of biologic agents in warfare is a recent occurrence, dating from the 1970s.
46. _____ Antibiotics provide effective treatment and prophylaxis for many bacterial illnesses if they are detected early.
47. _____ Aerosolized spread of a biologic agent is the most likely means of producing large numbers of victims.
48. _____ Anthrax is a viral agent.
49. _____ The most dangerous form of anthrax is inhalational anthrax.
50. _____ Inhalational anthrax can be spread person to person.
51. _____ MARK I kits contain autoinjectors with atropine and pralidoxime.
52. _____ MARK I kits are used to treat acute exposure to sulfur mustard.

53. _____ A patient exposed to cyanide gas has rapid respiratory and circulatory collapse and would be expected to exhibit signs of cyanosis.
54. _____ A good rule of thumb regarding exposure to cyanide gas is that if the victim can walk away from the vapor to fresh air, he or she may not need treatment.
55. _____ The clinical effects of mustard gas tend to be incapacitating rather than lethal.
56. _____ The clinical effects of mustard gas appear within 3 to 5 minutes after exposure.
57. _____ Phosgene liquid is toxic; the vapors formed do not pose a threat.
58. _____ Contamination is caused by radioactive particles that are physically present.
59. _____ Irradiation is caused by radioactive energy but is not physically present on the body.
60. _____ The contaminated victim can spread radioactive materials to others; the irradiated patient cannot.
61. _____ A dosimeter is a device worn by individuals that identifies the type of radiation and the rate of exposure.
62. _____ The dose of radiation absorbed at a distance of 10 feet is approximately one-fourth the dose that would be absorbed at 5 feet.
63. _____ Gamma rays pass through a victim and pose no threat to a rescuer once the patient is away from the radiation source.

CASE SCENARIO

Questions 64 to 68 refer to the following scenario.
You respond to a call for multiple people injured at the local shopping mall. On arrival you notice two people lying on the ground in front of the entrance to the mall. You and your partner put on full protective equipment. Approaching the scene, you notice at least 10 people lying on the floor inside the mall.

64. Your first priorities include:
   a. Entering the mall and performing a full assessment on each patient.
   b. Ensuring that a safe zone is established and calling for additional resources.
   c. Rapidly transporting the two patients outside the mall to the hospital, knowing that units arriving later will manage the scene.
   d. Immediately injecting yourself and your partner with a MARK I kit.

65. You begin to evaluate the two patients outside of the mall and determine that the patients have constricted pupils, muscle twitching, and secretions. Neither is responding to verbal or painful stimuli, and one begins to seize. Based on this clinical presentation, you suspect an exposure to:
   a. Cyanide gas
   b. Mustard gas
   c. Sulfur mustard
   d. A nerve agent

175

66. The first step in decontaminating the patient is to:
    a. Irrigate with water.
    b. Irrigate the patient with water and 1:100 dilution of chlorine.
    c. Remove the patient's clothes.
    d. No decontamination is needed because the patients are no longer directly exposed to the contaminant that is in the mall.

67. You call medical control and present the symptoms of your two patients while the hazardous materials team starts preparations to enter the mall. You would expect that medical control would instruct you to:
    a. Administer high-concentration oxygen and transport your patients.
    b. Administer a MARK I kit to each patient.
    c. Administer an EpiPen to the patient who is seizing.
    d. Immediately transport the patient who is not seizing; the other patient should be triaged as a "black" triage category.

68. Approximately 45 minutes after you arrive at the scene, the police inform you that they have received a call from someone claiming to have released sarin gas in the mall. Although this has not been confirmed, you know that if this is indeed the agent, the major threat of aerosolized sarin is:
    a. Contamination of the mucous membranes in exposed patients.
    b. Inhalation of the gas.
    c. Absorption through the skin requiring strict isolation precautions.
    d. Ingestion through contaminated food.

Chapter **30** **Weapons of Mass Destruction and the EMT**   Copyright © 2010, 2007, 2004, 1997, 1992 by Mosby, Inc., an affiliate of Elsevier Inc. All rights reserved.

31 Geriatric Emergencies

MULTIPLE CHOICE

1. The proportion of the population over age 65 is:
   a. Remaining the same.
   b. Decreasing.
   c. Increasing.
   d. Decreasing because of a shorter life expectancy.
2. You are treating a 75-year-old man named George Barns. The most appropriate way to refer to this patient is by calling him:
   a. Pops
   b. Grandpa
   c. George
   d. Mr. Barns
3. Elderly persons are more prone to dehydration because they:
   a. Tend to delay fluid intake, and their kidney function decreases with age.
   b. Tend to delay fluid intake, and their kidney function increases with age.
   c. Are more mobile and drink more often.
   d. Are less mobile and drink more often.
4. The highest rate of suicide is for:
   a. Men age 18 to 25 years
   b. Women age 18 to 25 years
   c. Men older than 65 years
   d. Women older than 65 years
5. An 82-year-old patient presents with visible bruises on her legs and back that appear to be in various stages of healing. You suspect:
   a. This is a normal condition of the aging process.
   b. She may be the victim of elder abuse.
   c. She has a bleeding disorder that requires hospital treatment.
   d. Blood clots caused by arteriosclerosis.

MATCHING

Questions 6-10. Match the physiologic parameters in column A with the expected change in column B.

Column A	Column B
6. _____ Stroke volume	a. Declines with age.
7. _____ Vital capacity	b. Increases with age.
8. _____ Residual volume	
9. _____ Maximum pulse rate	
10. _____ Resistance of blood vessels	

FILL IN THE BLANK

11. The total amount of air that can be moved in and out with a given breath is the _____ _____.
12. The amount of blood ejected from the heart with each beat is the _____ _____.
13. The amount of air that remains in the lungs at the end of an exhalation is the _____ _____.
14. Hardening of the arteries is called _____.
15. The decreased amount of bone density that occurs as a patient ages, particularly in women, is _____.

SHORT ANSWER

Questions 16-18. List three potential problems in the elderly patient that may make obtaining a history particularly difficult.

16. _____
    _____
17. _____
    _____
18. _____
    _____

Questions 19-22. List four potential conditions in the elderly patient that may result in a diminished or confused mental state.

19. _____
    _____
20. _____
    _____
21. _____
    _____
22. _____
    _____

Questions 23-25. List three signs that the EMT should check for when assessing a patient with suspected dehydration.

23. _____
    _____

177

24. _____

_____

25. _____

_____

TRUE/FALSE

26. _____ Elderly persons have a decreased ability to regulate their thermoregulatory system and therefore are more prone to environmental changes.

27. _____ The elderly population have had more diseases than the younger population and therefore are able to compensate more easily for severe illness.

28. _____ More than 90% of the deaths attributed to pneumonia and influenza occur in people older than 64 years.

29. _____ Drugs classified as beta blockers or calcium channel blockers may increase the patient's heart rate.

30. _____ If you encounter an elderly patient who has difficulty hearing, you should shout because this will compensate for the hearing impairment and enhance the patient's comprehension.

CASE SCENARIOS

Questions 31 to 33 are based on the following scenario.
You respond to a scene and encounter a 78-year-old woman who is sitting at her kitchen table. Her son called the ambulance because his mother "did not look right" and became very dizzy. On examination you determine that the patient was dizzy and sweaty, but now only complains of being a little weak. There are no neurologic deficits evident. The vital signs are pulse 88 beats/min and regular, blood pressure 142/80 mm Hg, and respiratory rate 14 breaths/min and normal. The patient is alert.

31. Based on your evaluation, you conclude that the patient:
    a. Has general malaise and is in no apparent distress.
    b. Is having an anaphylactic reaction and requires an EpiPen.
    c. May be having a heart attack even though she does not complain of chest pain.
    d. Is having a hypoglycemic episode and requires oral glucose.

32. Based on your evaluation, treatment would include:
    a. Transport in the position of comfort; no other interventions are needed.
    b. Administration of supplemental oxygen during transport.
    c. Administration of oral glucose, with a request for advanced life support intercept if available.
    d. The determination that the patient is stable at this time and does not need further evaluation at the hospital.

33. The patient tells you that she does not want to go to the hospital. You should:
    a. Allow the patient to sign a "refusal of medical aid" form.
    b. Attempt to convince the patient that hospital evaluation is needed; if she still refuses transportation, allow her to sign a "refusal of medical aid" form.
    c. Attempt to convince the patient that hospital evaluation is needed; if she still refuses transportation, restrain and transport.
    d. Attempt to convince the patient that hospital evaluation is needed; if she still refuses transportation, contact online medical direction in an attempt to have a physician convince the patient that hospital evaluation is needed.

Questions 34 and 35 refer to the following scenario.
You respond to the scene of a "man down" and encounter an 87-year-old man lying on the floor in his apartment. He tells you that he fell 2 days ago and has been unable to summon help until now. Your evaluation reveals a patient with pain in the left upper leg/hip area; his left leg appears to be outwardly rotated and slightly shorter than his right leg. There are good pulses, motor response, and sensation in all four extremities. The patient's vital signs are pulse 92 beats/min and regular/strong, blood pressure 168/88 mm Hg, and respiratory rate 16 breaths/min and regular, with full, equal bilateral breath sounds. The skin appears dry and "tents," and the patient has sunken eyes.

34. Based on the patient's clinical presentation, you would initiate treatment that includes:
    a. A traction splint applied to the left leg for a possible fractured femur.
    b. A long spine board and blankets to secure a possible hip fracture.
    c. An air splint to the left leg to treat a possible femur fracture.
    d. Application and inflation of the pneumatic anti-shock garment to treat a possible pelvic fracture.

35. The dry skin turgor and sunken eyes are indications of:
    a. Possible dehydration
    b. A physiologic response to pain
    c. The beginning stages of hypothermia
    d. Normal status in the elderly patient

Answer Key

Note: Numbers in parentheses indicate the page in the text where the question is discussed.

CHAPTER 1

1. a (2)
2. c (2)
3. c (2)
4. d (2)
5. b (3)
6. a (3)
7. a (3)
8. a (4)
9. c (8)
10. d (6)
11. a (9)
12. c (7)
13. d (16)
14. b (10)
15. b (14)
16. b (7)
17. a (8)
18. d (15)
19. c (16)
20. d (15)
21. d (16)
22. a (16)
23. b (7)
24. a (10-13)
25. b (10-13)

26. a (10-13)
27. a (10-13)
28. a (10-13)
29. a (10)
30. c (10)
31. c (10)
32. c (10)
33. lay rescuer (6)
34. dispatch (5)
35. Biotelemetry (6)
36. a. Reviewing prehospital documentation to ensure appropriate record keeping. (15)
    b. Reviewing ambulance runs to determine type of care provided and quality of care. (15)
    c. Gathering feedback from patients and hospital personnel on the quality of care. (15)
    d. Continuing education. (15)
    e. Performing preventive maintenance of the vehicle and equipment. (15)
    f. Maintaining personal skills. (15)
37. True (13)
38. False (13)
39. False (15)
40. True (15)
41. a (7)
42. Online (16)
43. d (10)

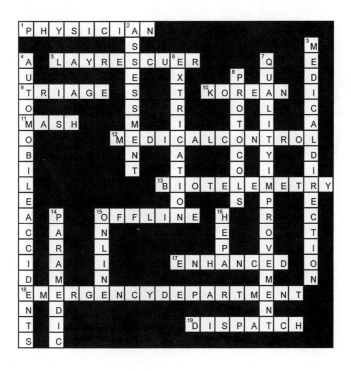

CHAPTER 2

1. a (41)
2. c (41)
3. c (45)
4. b (45)
5. b (45)
6. d (42)
7. b (42)
8. a (41)
9. d (41)
10. a (42)
11. d (22)
12. c (22)
13. a (26)
14. c (34)
15. a (23)
16. b (26)
17. d (26)
18. c (24)
19. d (40)
20. b (40)
21. b (22)
22. c (22)

23. b (30)
24. d (30)
25. c (30)
26. a (30)
27. chain of evidence (40)
28. communicable period (24)
29. depression (44)
30. immune (23)
31. incubation period (24)
32. Indirect contact (24)
33. microorganisms (23)
34. sharps container (35)
35. Standard precautions (26)
36. Tuberculosis (30)
37. vector borne (25)
38. a. There is little or no preexisting immunity in the human population. (37)
    b. It will cause illness in humans. (37)
    c. It has the potential for sustained transmission from person to person. (37)

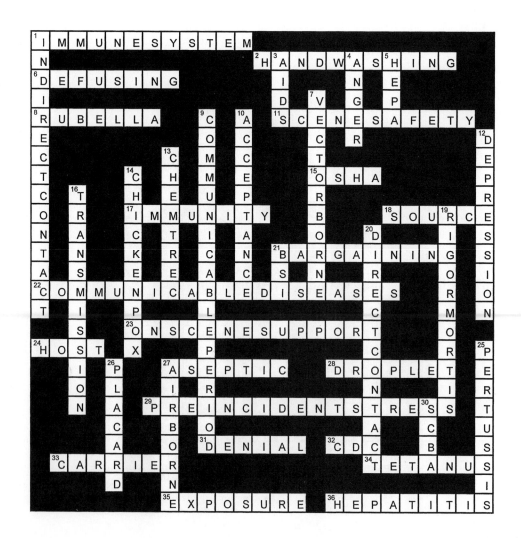

CHAPTER 3

1. b (51)
2. c (52)
3. b (54)
4. b (54)
5. c (55)
6. b (56)
7. c (56)
8. a (56)
9. d (55)
10. a (60)
11. c (59)
12. a (54)
13. b (56)
14. c (55)
15. b (60)
16. standard of care (53)
17. battery (56)
18. Duty to act (54)
    Breach of duty (54)
    Injury (54)
    Causal connection (54)
19. c (56)
20. b (55)
21. c (54)
22. a (53)
23. c (58)
24. b (59)

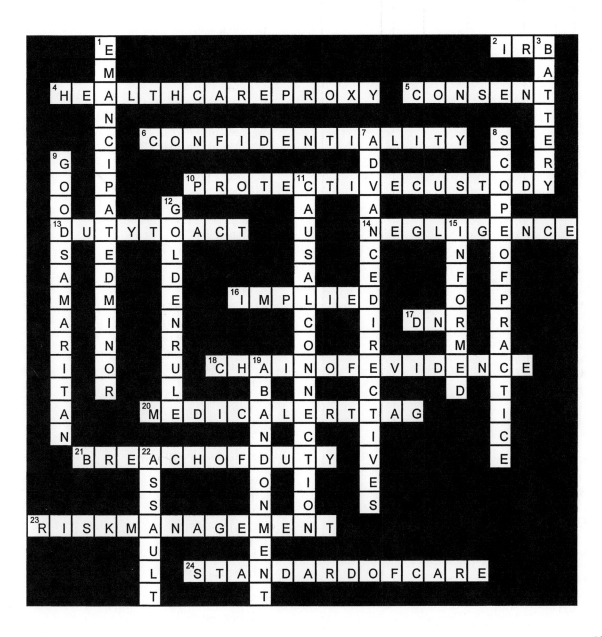

CHAPTER 4

1. a (66)
2. a (69)
3. c (66)
4. c (72)
5. b (72)
6. c (72)
7. d (80)
8. b (80)
9. d (87)
10. a (88)
11. a (84)
12. b (92)
13. c (84)
14. d (70)
15. d (95)
16. c (97)
17. c (97)
18. c (98)
19. b (99)
20. a (99)
21. a (95)
22. b (67)
23. e (67)
24. f (67)
25. a (67)
26. c (67)
27. d (67)
28. c (71)
29. a (71)
30. e (71)
31. b (71)
32. d (71)
33. a (74)
34. c (74)
35. b (74)
36. Anterior (67)
37. Arteries (67)
38. Bilateral (67)
39. Cartilage (69)
40. Dermis (96)
41. diaphragm (71)
42. kidneys (99)
43. Larynx (80)
44. Ligaments (70)
45. radial artery (89)
46. Tendons (70)
47. Thorax (71)
48. Trachea (72)
49. Veins (88)
50. b (67)
51. d (67)
52. b (74)
53. d (71)
54. b (80)
55. d (85)
56. c (86)
57. d (91)
58. epinephrine (adrenaline) (97)
59. a. Extension (68)
    b. Flexion (68)
60. a. Skull (70)
    b. Manubrium (70)
    c. Clavicle (70)
    d. Sternum (70)
    e. Xiphoid process (70)
    f. Ribs (70)
    g. Radius (70)
    h. Ulna (70)
    i. Pelvis (70)
    j. Iliac crest (70)
    k. Ischium (70)
    l. Pubis (70)
    m. Carpals (70)
    n. Metacarpals (70)
    o. Phalanges (70)
    p. Femur (70)
    q. Patella (70)
    r. Tibia (70)
    s. Fibula (70)
    t. Tarsals (70)
    u. Metatarsals (70)
    v. Phalanges (70)
    w. Humerus (70)
    x. Cervical vertebrae (70)
    y. Thoracic vertebrae (70)
    z. Coccyx (70)
61. a. Frontal bone (71)
    b. Parietal bone (71)
    c. Nasal bone (71)
    d. Mandible (71)
    e. Temporal bone (71)
    f. Orbital bones (71)
    g. Zygomatic bone (71)
    h. Maxilla (71)
62. a. Right atrium (87)
    b. Tricuspid valve (87)
    c. Right ventricle (87)
    d. Pulmonary valve (87)
    e. Aortic valve (87)
    f. Left atrium (87)
    g. Mitral valve (87)
    h. Left ventricle (87)
    i. Ventricular septum (87)
63. a. Cerebrum (95)
    b. Corpus collosum (95)
    c. Thalamus (95)
    d. Midbrain (95)
    e. Cerebellum (95)
    f. Brain stem (95)
    g. Medulla (95)
    h. Pons (95)
    i. Pituitary gland (95)
    j. Hypothalamus (95)
64. a. Hair shaft (97)
    b. Sweat pore (97)
    c. Epidermis (97)

d. Dermis (97)
e. Hypodermis (97)
f. Hair follicle (97)
g. Sweat gland (97)
h. Nerve fiber (97)
i. Sebaceous (oil) gland (97)
65. a. Mouth (98)
b. Liver (98)
c. Gallbladder (98)
d. Large intestine (98)
e. Small intestine (98)
f. Salivary glands (98)
g. Pharynx (98)
h. Esophagus (98)

i. Stomach (98)
j. Diaphragm (98)
k. Pancreas (98)
l. Rectum (98)
66. a. Urinary bladder (99)
b. Vena cava (99)
c. Abdominal aorta (99)
d. Adrenal gland (99)
e. Kidney (99)
f. Ureter (99)
g. Urethra (99)

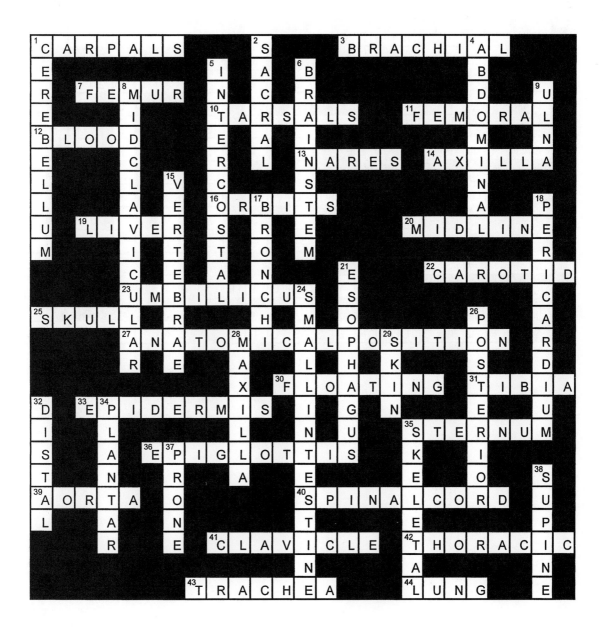

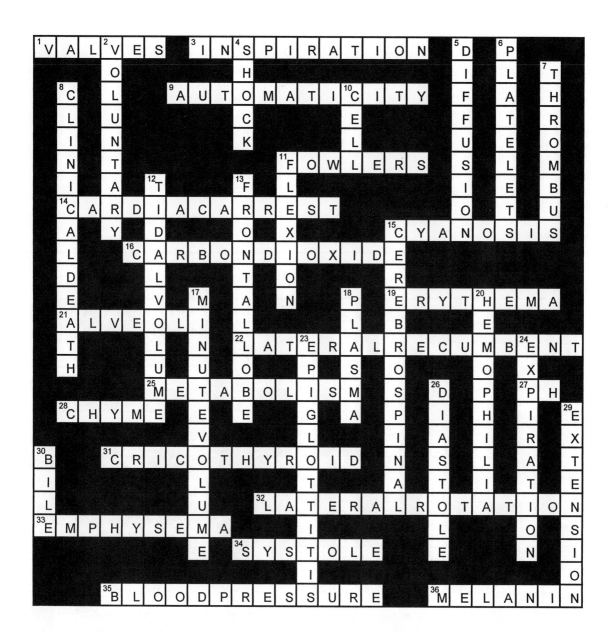

CHAPTER 5

1. b (106)
2. c (106)
3. c (107)
4. a (107)
5. c (107)
6. a (107)
7. a (108)
8. c (108)
9. b (108)
10. a (Chapter 24)
11. b (Chapter 24)
12. b (108)
13. b (109)
14. left lateral recumbent (114)
15. clothes drag (109)
16. airway (114)
17. f (111, 112)
18. d (111, 112)
19. g (111, 112)
20. b (111, 112)
21. c (111, 112)
22. a (111, 112)
23. e (111, 112)
24. a (112)
25. b (112)
26. c (112)
27. d (111)
28. c (112)
29. c, a, e, b, d (116, 117)

CHAPTER 6

1. b (133)
2. b (133)
3. a (134)
4. a (136)
5. c (136)
6. d (134)
7. b (135)
8. d (136)
9. b (145)
10. d (151)
11. a (136)
12. b (133)
13. c (147)
14. c (140)
15. a (141)
16. c (138)
17. c (141)
18. a (156)
19. a (155)
20. d (143)
21. b (144)
22. d (144)
23. d (146)
24. c (145)
25. b (146)
26. a (146)

27. c (146)
28. b (146)
29. a (141)
30. a (141)
31. c (141)
32. b (152)
33. a (143)
34. b (145)
35. a (157)
36. b (147)
37. b (148)
38. a (148)
39. minute volume (136)
40. nasal septum (131)
41. cyanosis (140)
42. hypoxemia (148)
43. cricoid pressure (144)
44. cricoid cartilage (149)
45. b (142)
46. a (157)
47. d (143)
48. c (136)
49. d (138)
50. c (151)
51. b (151, 152)
52. b (152)
53. a (152)
54. c (Chapter 4)
55. b (141)
56. c (140)
57. c (143)
58. a (146)
59. d, b, a, c, e, f (165)

CHAPTER 7

1. a (208)
2. a (195)
3. c (195)
4. b (187)
5. d (187)
6. c (193)
7. a (194)
8. c (194)
9. a (214)
10. a (197)
11. b (197)
12. b (198)
13. b (198)
14. c (206)
15. b (192)
16. b (195)
17. d (185)
18. a (185)
19. d (185)
20. a (198)
21. b (198)
22. a (198)
23. a (196)

24. c (187)
25. b (173)
26. d (174)
27. a (174)
28. a (174)
29. c (174)
30. a (175)
31. c (175)
32. b (172)
33. a (172)
34. d (177)
35. b (180)
36. c (210)
37. b (182)
38. a (186)
39. d (183)
40. a (208)
41. a (195)
42. c (195)
43. c (194)
44. d (185)
45. d (182)
46. a (183)
47. b (183)
48. a (186)
49. d (184)
50. b (184)
51. a (195)
52. a (195)
53. c (196)
54. d (199)
55. c (187)
56. d
57. c (193)
58. a (194)
59. a (197)
60. d (204)
61. c (204)
62. d (204)
63. d (199)
64. a (203)
65. b (204)
66. a (204)
67. a (195)
68. b (194)
69. c (206)
70. b (199)
71. c (206)
72. d (199)
73. c (206)
74. d (187, 189)
75. c (187)
76. c (207)
77. b (190)
78. a (190)
79. d (200)
80. d (192)
81. b (191)
82. a (192)

83. d (192)
84. d (192)
85. b (192)
86. a (206)
87. d (206)
88. c (207)
89. d (185)
90. b (207)
91. a (207)
92. a (206)
93. b (217)
94. d (207)
95. b (183)
96. a (183)
97. c (183)
98. d (183)
99. blood pressure (197)
100. conjunctiva (221)
101. 3 (198)
102. SAMPLE (187)
103. nasal flaring (193)
104. Retractions (193)
105. Multiple-casualty incident (180)
106. Dislocation (205)
107. Jugular vein distention (204)
108. mechanism of injury (177)
109. DCAP/BTLS (200)
110. paradoxical motion or flail chest (204)
111. tracheal deviation (204)
112. Onset (189)
113. Provocation (189)
114. Quality (189)
115. Radiation (189)
116. Severity (189)
117. Time (189)
118. Abdominal pain (189)
119. constrict (204)
120. skull fracture (204)
121. forward (Chapter 20)
122. AVPU (182)
123. chest expansion (208)
124. older adults (208)
125. Are you pregnant? (192)
126. How long have you been pregnant? (192)
127. Do you have any pain or contractions? (192)
128. Do you have any vaginal bleeding or discharge? (192)
129. Do you feel the need to push? (192)
130. When was your last menstrual period? (192)
131. How do you feel? (192)
132. Ask appropriate questions to determine suicidal tendencies (e.g., Do you want to hurt or kill yourself?) (192)
133. Is the patient a threat to self or others? (192)
134. Is there a medical problem along with the behavioral emergency? (192)
135. Has the patient/family undertaken any interventions? (192)
136. What was the substance involved? (192)

137. When did the patient ingest the substance or become exposed? (192)
138. How much of the substance was ingested? (192)
139. Over what period of time was the substance ingested? (192)
140. What, if any, interventions have already occurred? (192)
141. What is the patient's estimated weight? (192)
142. Can the patient or bystander describe the event? (192)
143. What was the onset of the event (what was the patient doing when the event began)? (192)
144. How long has this been going on? (192)
145. Are there any associated symptoms present? (192)
146. Is there any evidence of trauma? (192)
147. What, if any, interventions have already occurred? (192)
148. Has the patient had a seizure? (192)
149. Does the patient have a fever? (192)
150. Does the patient have a history of allergies? (192)
151. What was the patient exposed to? (192)
152. How was the patient exposed? (192)
153. What have been the effects of the exposure? (192)
154. What has been the progression (speed of onset, specific complaints) of the exposure? (192)
155. What, if any, interventions have already occurred? (192)
156. What was the source of the environmental emergency? (192)
157. What was the environment in which the exposure occurred? (192)
158. What was the duration of the exposure? (192)
159. Did the patient lose consciousness? (192)
160. What effects, general or local, has the patient experienced? (192)

161. Repeat the initial (primary) assessment (206)
162. Repeat taking the vital signs (206)
163. Repeat the focused (secondary) assessment (206)
164. Check on all interventions that have been made
165. Pale skin from shock (195)
166. Cyanotic skin from inadequate oxygenation (195)
167. Flushed skin from fever (195)
168. True (172)
169. False (172)
170. True (172)
171. False (175)
172. False (176)
173. True (177)
174. False (180)
175. False (174)
176. False (180)
177. False (199)
178. True (199)
179. True
180. False (200)
181. True (209)
182. b (173)
183. b (182)
184. d (207)
185. c (181)
186. d (187)
187. a (199)
188. c (182)
189. c (200)
190. c (190)
191. d (196)
192. d (206)
193. c (191)

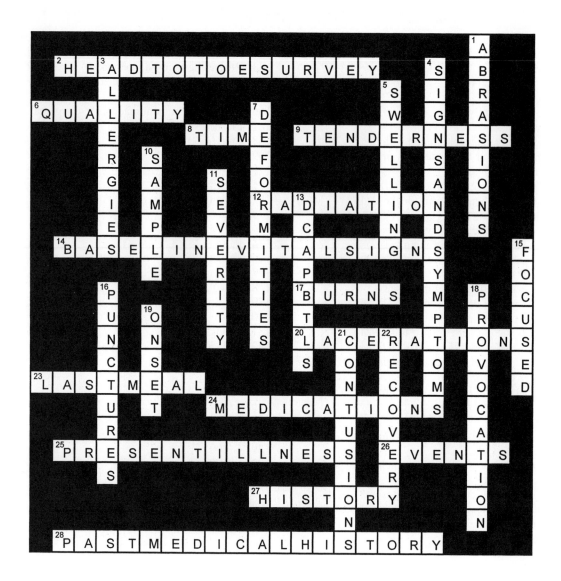

Across:
2. HEADTOTOESURVEY
6. QUALITY
8. TIME
9. TENDERNESS
12. RADIATION
14. BASELINEVITALSIGNS
17. BURNS
20. LACERATIONS
23. LASTMEAL
24. MEDICATIONS
25. PRESENTILLNESS
26. EVENTS
27. HISTORY
28. PASTMEDICALHISTORY

CHAPTER 8

1. d (230)
2. a (230)
3. b (230)
4. d (230)
5. b (231)
6. b (231)
7. a (231)
8. c (231)
9. b (230)
10. a (230)
11. b (230)
12. c (229)
13. d (231)
14. b (230)
15. c (234)
16. c (234)
17. Treat with special respect. (233)
18. Move elderly patients with extra care. (233)
19. Be sensitive to the spouse's concerns. (233)
20. Allow the parent to accompany the child. (234)
21. Bring along objects that help make the child feel more secure. (233)
22. Interact with both the parent and the child. (234)
23. Be honest with the child. (234)
24. If the patient can read lips, look directly at his or her face and speak in a normal, slow voice. (234)
25. Uses short written questions as necessary. (234)
26. Be patient. (234)
27. Explain to the patient what you are doing. (234)
28. Maintain physical contact with the blind patient. (234)
29. Describe in detail what you are doing. (234)
30. If the patient has a support dog, bring the dog with the patient or arrange for care of the dog. (234)
31. Use simple terms. (234)
32. Give simple explanations. (234)
33. Reinforce orientation and simple explanations. (234)
34. Allow the patient ample time to respond to questions. (234)
35. Assume that the patient can understand what you are saying. (234)
36. Give simple explanations and reinforcement. (234)
37. Determine the capability of the patient to understand. (234)
38. Distinguish mental from physical disability. (234)
39. Assume that the patient can understand what you are saying. (234)
40. a (230)
41. repeater (236)
42. d (229)

CHAPTER 9

1. a (228)
2. b (240)
3. a (245)
4. d (246)
5. a (246)
6. c (245)
7. c (243)
8. b (243)
9. b (241)
10. a (250)
11. a (241, 242)
12. a (247)
13. c (247)
14. d (240)
15. b (247)
16. a (250)
17. d (241)
18. d (241)
19. b (248)
20. ♂ (242)
21. ♀ (242)
22. $\bar{a}$ (242)
23. BP (242)
24. $\bar{c}$ (242)
25. c/o (242)
26. CPR (242)
27. DOB (242)
28. Hx (242)
29. LLQ (242)
30. LUQ (242)
31. NTG (242)
32. O_2 (242)
33. po (242)
34. Pt (242)
35. Px (242)
36. RLQ (242)
37. RUQ (242)
38. SL (242)
39. SOB (242)
40. Tx (242)
41. y/o (242)
42. b (243)
43. c (250)

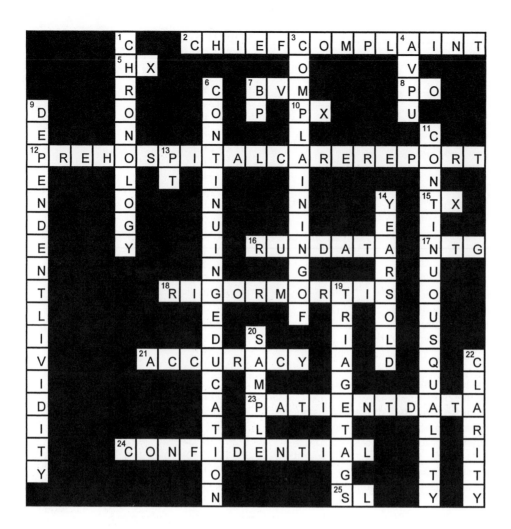

CHAPTER 10

1. a (255)
2. d (256)
3. c (257)
4. b (258)
5. c (258)
6. d (257)
7. b (260)
8. c (263)
9. d (257)
10. a (257)
11. e (257)
12. b (257)
13. c (257)
14. a (257)
15. b (257)
16. b (257)
17. b (257)
18. b (257)
19. a (257)
20. a (257)
21. pharmacology (255)
22. medication (drug) (255)
23. 10 kg (258)
24. activated charcoal (257)
25. 1000 (257)
26. Right patient (262)
27. Right drug (262)
28. Right dose (262)
29. Right route of administration (262)
30. Right time of administration (262)
31. b (258)
32. c
33. d (257)
34. a (257)
35. c (258)
36. d (258)

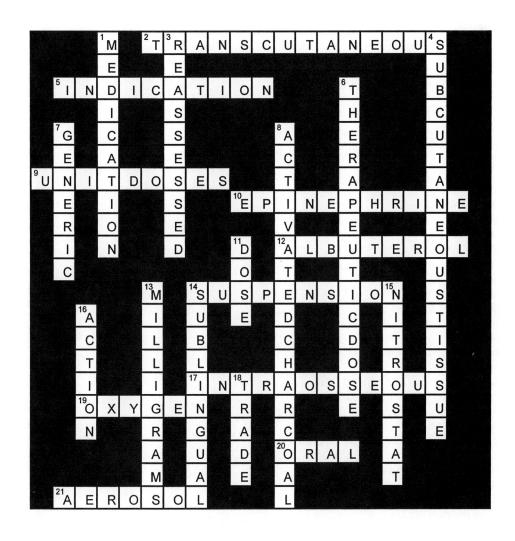

CHAPTER 11

1. b (266)
2. b (266)
3. a (266)
4. a (268)
5. c (266)
6. d (266)
7. d (268)
8. b (145, Chapter 6)
9. c (279)
10. c (272)
11. b (266)
12. a (272)
13. a (268)
14. b (268)
15. c (270)
16. d (270)
17. c (165, Chapter 6)
18. c (165, Chapter 6)
19. d (268)
20. a (276)
21. b (271)
22. d (276)
23. a (279)
24. b (280)
25. a (280)
26. c (215)
27. a (274)
28. b (274)
29. b (274)
30. b (274)
31. b (274)
32. a (274)
33. tripod (270)
34. minute volume (268)
35. pink puffer (277)
36. pneumonia (279)
37. hyperventilation syndrome (279)
38. AVPU (270)
39. 12 times per minute (271, 272)
40. 20 times per minute (271)
41. 20 times per minute (271)
42. Onset: What were you doing when the symptoms began? (272)
43. Provocation: Does anything make your breathing problem worse? (272)
44. Quality: Is there any associated pain? If there is, where is the pain, can you point to it with one finger, how would you describe it, and does the pain get worse when you breathe? (272)
45. Radiation: If you do have pain, does the pain go anywhere, such as to your arm, neck, or jaw?
46. Severity: How severe is the shortness of breath (or the pain)? Can you rate it on a scale of 1 to 10? (272)
47. Time: How long have you had the respiratory distress and/or the pain? (272)
48. d (273)
49. c (279)

50. a (278
51. d (268)
52. a (276)
53. c (277)
54. d (278)
55. c (278)
56. b (278)
57. d, i, e, f, a, g, b, h (282, 283)

CHAPTER 12

1. d (287)
2. c (291)
3. c (289)
4. b (290)
5. a (289)
6. d (289)
7. b (291)
8. b (290)
9. c (289)
10. b (291)
11. a (291)
12. b (290)
13. c (290)
14. a (293)
15. b (293)
16. b (298, 299)
17. d (297)
18. a (293)
19. b (293)
20. c (293)
21. b (293)
22. d (295)
23. c (297)
24. b (295)
25. b (295)
26. b (296)
27. a (297)
28. c (297)
29. a (288)
30. d (297)
31. a (294)
32. c (297)
33. c (297)
34. d (295)
35. b (295)
36. d (293)
37. b (288)
38. b (296)
39. b (288)
40. b (309)
41. c (306)
42. c (316)
43. a (317)
44. b (287)
45. b (310)
46. c (307)
47. c (310)
48. a (310)

49. a (303)
50. a (307)
51. a (303)
52. b (307, 308)
53. c (287, 303)
54. a (303)
55. c (303)
56. c (287, 303)
57. b (288)
58. b (310)
59. b (297)
60. b (309)
61. c (309)
62. b (299)
63. a (299)
64. b (299)
65. a (299)
66. a (299)
67. Allergies to aspirin (299)
68. Recently taken aspirin (299)
69. Recent history of gastrointestinal bleeding (299)
70. Onset: What were you doing when the symptoms began? (295)
71. Provocation: Does anything make the pain better or worse? (295)
72. Quality: How would you describe the pain? (295)
73. Radiation: Does the pain go anywhere, such as to your arm, neck, or jaw? (295)
74. Severity: Describe the pain on a scale of 1 to 10 and compare it with previous episodes, if appropriate. (295)
75. Time: How long have you had the pain? (295)
76. Early access to 9-1-1 (287)
77. Early CPR (287)
78. Early defibrillation (287)
79. Early advanced care (287)
80. Nausea (295)
81. Vomiting (295)
82. Weakness (295)
83. Shortness of breath (295)
84. Palpitations (295)
85. Lightheadedness (295)
86. Sweating (295)
87. Dizziness (295)
88. Loss of consciousness (295)
89. c (297)
90. b (303)
91. d (298, 299)
92. c (299)
93. a (295)
94. a (297)
95. d (301)
96. f, b, e, c, d, a (314, 315)

CHAPTER 13

1. d (327)
2. b (329)
3. d (328)
4. a (327)
5. c (327)
6. c (324, 327)
7. c (328)
8. b (327)
9. b (329)
10. b (327)
11. b (327)
12. b (327)
13. a (329)
14. c
15. c (337)
16. b (328, 329)
17. a (328, 329)
18. a (328, 329)
19. b (328, 329)
20. a (328, 329)
21. a (328, 329)
22. b (328, 329)
23. b (328, 329)
24. transient ischemic attack (332)
25. Hypertension (332)
26. cerebrovascular accident (332)
27. embolism (332)
28. thrombus (333)
29. Alcohol withdrawal (330)
30. Drug withdrawal (330)
31. Eclampsia (toxemia of pregnancy) (330)
32. Epilepsy (330)
33. Fever (330)
34. Hypoglycemia (330)
35. Hypoxia (330)
36. Infections (330)
37. Poisonings (330)
38. Trauma (330)
39. False (332, 333)
40. False (332, 333)
41. True (332, 333)
42. True (332, 333)
43. False (332, 333)
44. True (332, 333)
45. False (332, 333)
46. d (323)
47. d (332)
48. b (334)
49. b (334)
50. b (330)
51. c (330)
52. c (331)

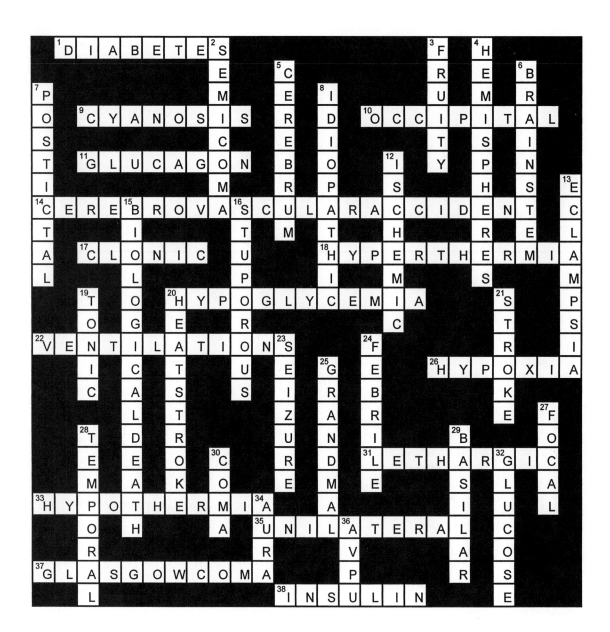

CHAPTER 14

1. a (352)
2. c (351)
3. b (351)
4. c (354)
5. c (353)
6. b (353)
7. a (354)
8. a (354)
9. c (355)
10. c (355, 358)
11. c (356)
12. b (352)
13. d (353)
14. d (352)
15. b (352)
16. a (352)
17. c (352)
18. Consult medical direction for the possibility of a second injection of epinephrine. (352)
19. to 28. Ten of the following 20:
    Abdominal pain (352)
    Anxiety (352)
    Coughing (352)
    Cramping (352)
    Diarrhea (352)
    Facial edema (352)
    Fainting (352)
    Hoarseness (352)
    Itching (352)
    Itchy and watery eyes (352)
    Laryngeal edema (352)
    Loss of voice (352)
    Pharyngeal edema (352)
    Runny nose (352)
    Sense of impending doom (352)
    Sneezing (352)
    Tightness in throat (352)
    Tingling feeling (352)
    Vomiting (352)
    Wheezing (352)
29. to 38. Ten of the following 16:
    Cardiac arrest (352, 354)
    Decreased mental state (352, 354)
    Difficulty breathing (352, 354)
    Flushing of skin (352, 354)
    Hives (352, 354)
    Hypotension (352, 354)
    Rapid, labored breathing (352, 354)
    Rapid pulse (352, 354)
    Respiratory arrest (352, 354)
    Stridor and noisy breathing (352, 354)
    Swelling of face (352, 354)
    Swelling of feet (352, 354)
    Swelling of hands (352, 354)
    Swelling of neck (352, 354)
    Swelling of tongue (352, 354)
    Wheezing (352, 354)

39. Does the patient have a history of allergies? (356)
40. What was the patient exposed to? (356)
41. How was the patient exposed? (356)
42. What have been the effects of the exposure? (356)
43. What has been the progression (speed of onset, specific complaints) of the exposure? (356)
44. What, if any, interventions have already occurred? (356)
45. Chest pain (355)
46. Dizziness (355)
47. Excitability and anxiousness (355)
48. Headache (355)
49. Increased heart rate (355)
50. Nausea (355)
51. Pallor (355)
52. Vomiting (355)
53. d (355)
54. c (355)
55. c (355)
56. d (356)
57. c (355)
58. a (351)

CHAPTER 15

1. c (364)
2. b (366)
3. d (366)
4. c (367)
5. c (367)
6. d (369)
7. c (369)
8. d (369)
9. a (369)
10. d (369)
11. a (371)
12. d (364)
13. c (363)
14. a (363)
15. d (363)
16. b (363)
17. c (364)
18. e (364)
19. d (364)
20. a (364)
21. b (364)
22. Ethylene glycol (370)
23. Methanol (370)
24. 800-222-1222 (363)
25. What was the substance involved? (365, 366)
26. When did the patient ingest or become exposed? (365, 366)
27. How much of the substance was ingested? (365, 366)
28. Over what period of time was the substance ingested? (365, 366)
29. What, if any, interventions have already occurred? (365, 366)
30. What is the patient's estimated weight? (365, 366)

31. What effects, if any, has the patient experienced since the ingestion/exposure? (365, 366)
32. b (369)
33. c (362)
34. b (366)
35. b (371)
36. c (373)
37. a (373)
38. a (373)
39. c (366, 369)
40. d (366)
41. a (367)
42. c (364, 366)
43. b (373)
44. d (373)
45. c (362)
46. b (375, 376)
47. d
48. b (369)

CHAPTER 16

1. a (385)
2. d (386)
3. b (386)
4. c (386)
5. a (387)
6. d (386)
7. c (387, 388)
8. c (385)
9. a (385)
10. b (388)
11. d (387)
12. b (395)
13. b (395)
14. b (389)
15. b (389)
16. d (394)
17. a (396)
18. b (387)
19. c (389)
20. a (385)
21. a (386, 389)
22. c (390)
23. c (393)
24. b (395)
25. a (391)
26. c (391)
27. d (391)
28. c (391)
29. a (392)
30. b (391)
31. c (392)
32. d (392)
33. a (392)
34. a (393)
35. b (393)
36. c (399)
37. a (399)
38. a (390)
39. b (390)
40. d (390)
41. c (394)
42. c (394)
43. b (394)
44. a (390)
45. c (390)
46. c (390)
47. a (390)
48. b (390)
49. b (390)
50. c (390)
51. a (390)
52. b (390)
53. a (390)
54. b (390)
55. b (390)
56. b (390)
57. b (399, 400)
58. d (399, 400)
59. a (399, 400)
60. c (399, 400)
61. What was the source of the environmental emergency? (388)
62. What was the environment that the exposure occurred in? (388)
63. What was the duration of the exposure? (388)
64. Did the patient lose consciousness? (388)
65. What effects, general or local, has the patient experienced? (388)
66. False (394)
67. False (394)
68. True (397)
69. True (397)
70. True (397)
71. False (397)
72. c (373)
73. c (391)
74. b (391)
75. a (393)
76. b (394)
77. d (391)
78. b (394)
79. b (394)
80. c (394)
81. c (394)
82. d (394)
83. a (394)
84. c (394)
85. d (390)
86. a (391)
87. b (397)
88. d (397)
89. b (397)
90. a (399)
91. c (399)

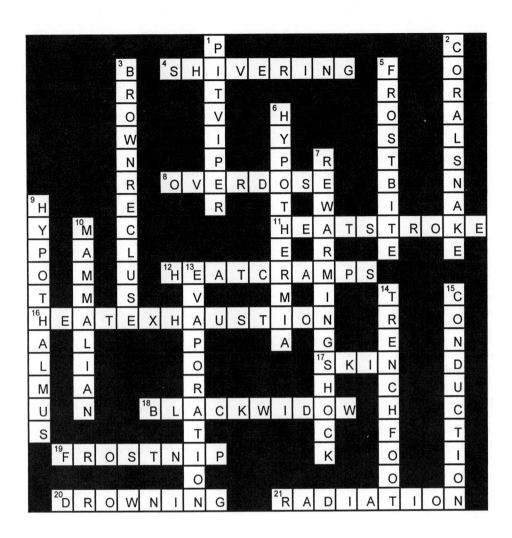

197

CHAPTER 17

1. d (411)
2. b (416)
3. a (410)
4. a (410)
5. c (410)
6. a (410)
7. b (411)
8. c (412)
9. c (412)
10. b (416)
11. a (415)
12. b (416)
13. c (410)
14. d (410)
15. b (409)
16. a (418)
17. How do you feel? (417)
18. Ask appropriate questions to determine suicidal tendencies. (417)
19. Is the patient a threat to self or others? (417)
20. Is there a medical problem along with the behavioral emergency? (417)
21. What is the patient's past medical history? (417)
22. Has the patient/family undertaken any interventions? (417)
23. What medications does the patient take, and does he or she take them as prescribed? (417)
24. Excessive cold (409)
25. Excessive heat (409)
26. Head trauma (409)
27. Inadequate blood flow to the brain (shock, stroke) (409)
28. Low blood oxygen level (409)
29. Low blood sugar level (409)
30. Mind-altering substances (409)
31. Psychogenic, resulting in psychotic thinking, depression, or panic (409)
32. True (411)
33. False (411)
34. False (412)
35. True (416)
36. True (413)
37. b (410)
38. b (416)
39. c (413)
40. a (413)
41. a (410)
42. a (416)
43. a (410)
44. c (411)
45. d (410)

CHAPTER 18

1. a (428)
2. d (428)
3. Tension phase (424)

4. Violence phase (424)
5. Honeymoon ("wine and roses") phase (424)
6. Multiple bruises in different stages of healing (425)
7. Patterned bruised (425)
8. Black eyes, lacerations, welts (425)
9. Defensive injuries to the arms (425)
10. Broken bones (425)
11. Burns (425)
12. Cuts or open wounds (425)
13. Sprains, dislocations, internal injuries (425)
14. Broken eyeglasses (425)
15. Signs of restraint (425)
16. "Prone to accidents" (425)
17. Multiple calls to the person's home (425)
18. Signs of insecurity (427)
19. Poor self-esteem (427)
20. Destructive behavior (427)
21. Angry acts (e.g., starting fires, cruelty to animals) (427)
22. Withdrawal (427)
    or
    Poor development of basic skills (427)
    Alcohol or drug abuse (427)
    Suicide (427)
23. Untreated wounds (427, 428)
24. Poor personal hygiene (427, 428)
25. Untreated medical conditions (427, 428)
26. Unsanitary living conditions (427, 428)
27. Harmful living conditions (427, 428)
28. Failure to thrive (427, 428)
29. Weight loss (427, 428)
30. Constant demand for attention from EMT (427, 428)
31. False (424)
32. False (424)
33. False
34. True (424)
35. False (424)
36. False (425)
37. b (427)
38. c (427)

CHAPTER 19

1. a (434)
2. c (434)
3. b (438)
4. b (435)
5. b (436)
6. b (438)
7. a (438)
8. b (442)
9. b (443)
10. c (443)
11. b (446)
12. b (450)
13. c (444)
14. b (445)
15. b (444)
16. b (446)

17. b (446)
18. a (446)
19. b (447)
20. b (446, 447)
21. a (446)
22. b
23. b (446)
24. c (436)
25. d (436)
26. d (436)
27. a (440)
28. a (448)
29. d (446)
30. c (452)
31. b (450)
32. c (450)
33. b (437)
34. b (437)
35. c (454)
36. c (441)
37. d (434, 441)
38. a (442)
39. a (448)
40. c (451)
41. 5 minutes (447)
42. ½ inch (447)
43. 20 to 30 mL (446)
44. Are you pregnant? (440)
45. How long have you been pregnant? (440)
46. Do you have any pain or contractions? (440)
47. Do you have any vaginal bleeding or discharge? (440)
48. Do you feel the need to push? (440)
49. When was your last menstrual period? (440)

50. Is the baby crowning? (440)
51. Ruptured ectopic pregnancy (454)
52. Ruptured ovarian cyst (454)
53. Pale color (447)
54. Retractions (447)
55. Grunting (447)
56. Nasal flaring (447)
57. Appearance (color) (447)
58. Pulse (heart rate) (447)
59. Grimace (vigorous cry on stimulation) (447)
60. Activity (extremities: good tone, flexed, moving) (447)
61. Respirations (447)
62. b (451)
63. b (451)
64. b (451)
65. b (454, Chapter 18)
66. b (454, Chapter 18)
67. c (452)
68. b (453)
69. a (453)
70. c (453)
71. b (449)
72. b (449)
73. a (447)
74. b (447)
75. b
76. c (440)
77. b (446)
78. a (446)
79. c (438)
80. b (451)

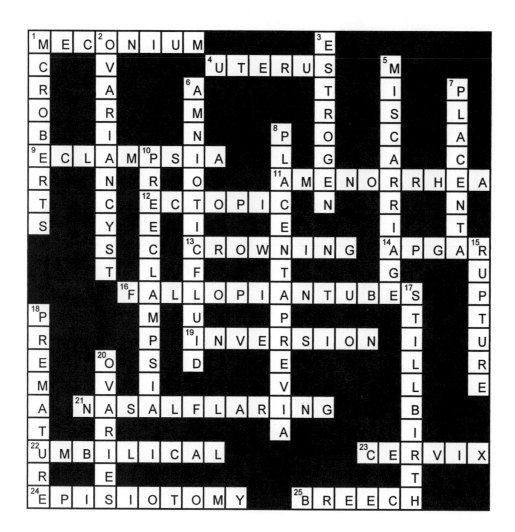

CHAPTER 20

1. b (461)
2. b (462)
3. c (462)
4. a (469)
5. a (471)
6. d (470)
7. b (463)
8. d (464)
9. b (464)
10. d (461)
11. b (461)
12. d (466)
13. a (466)
14. a (470)
15. d (471)
16. c (471)
17. a (473)
18. d (472)
19. c (473)
20. a (472, 473)
21. c (475)
22. d (473)
23. a (467)
24. d (463)
25. stroke volume (461)
26. cardiac output (461)
27. heart rate (461)
28. blood pressure (462)
29. False (472)
30. True (471)
31. False
32. False
33. True (469)
34. False (464)
35. True (467)
36. c (464)
37. d (466)
38. a (461)
39. d (470)
40. b (470)
41. d (469)
42. b (469)
43. b (471)
44. c (471)
45. a (471)
46. c (467)
47. d (469)
48. b (464)
49. d (465)
50. b (466)
51. a

CHAPTER 21

1. c (479)
2. a (479)
3. c (479)
4. d (479)
5. c (479)
6. b (479)
7. a (485)
8. b (485)
9. b (486)
10. b (486)
11. b (488)
12. a (498, 505)
13. a (489)
14. b (489)
15. d (489)
16. b (489)
17. a (489)
18. b (489)
19. c (489)
20. b (490)
21. b (490)
22. c (490, 491)
23. b (500)
24. a (501)
25. c (491)
26. a (492)
27. c (492)
28. c (492)
29. a (492)
30. b (493)
31. a (485)
32. d (485)
33. b (495)
34. c (495)
35. b (495)
36. b (496)
37. c (496)
38. b (496)
39. c (497)
40. a (498)
41. b (499)
42. b (499)
43. d (498)
44. c (498)
45. c (499)
46. c (498)
47. c (499)
48. b (500)
49. b (500)
50. b (501)
51. a (501)
52. c (501)
53. a (501)
54. c (501)
55. b (501)
56. d (501)
57. c (501)
58. a (501)
59. d (501)
60. c (501)
61. a (496)
62. e (481)
63. c (481)

64. d (481)
65. a (481)
66. b (481)
67. c (487)
68. a (487)
69. d (487)
70. b (487)
71. b (497, 498)
72. c (497, 498)
73. a (497, 498)
74. f (497, 498)
75. e (497, 498)
76. d (497, 498)
77. 5 (499, 500)
78. 3 (499, 500)
79. 2 (499, 500)
80. 4 (499, 500)
81. 1 (499, 500)
82. 55 (499, 500)
83. 5 (499, 500)
84. Singed nasal hairs (498)
85. Sputum with black particles (carbonaceous sputum) (498)
86. Burns around the mouth and nose (498)
87. Hoarseness of voice (498)
88. Respiratory distress (498)
89. a (488)
90. c (488)
91. b (490, 491)
92. b (490, 491)
93. b (481, 485)
94. a (481, 485)
95. c (488)
96. b (493)
97. c (492)
98. b (499-501)
99. d (499-501)
100. b (499-501)
101. c (497, 498)
102. b (496)
103. b (499)
104. b (499)
105. a (501-503)
106. c (501-503)
107. b (501-503)
108. c (501-503)
109. a, c, b (506, 507)
110. b, c, a (509)

CHAPTER 22

1. c (515)
2. c (515)
3. b (515)
4. a (515)
5. b (515)
6. c (515)
7. a (515)
8. c (515)
9. b (515)
10. d (515)
11. c (516)
12. b (516)
13. c (516)
14. d (517)
15. c (518, 519)
16. a (521)
17. c (525)
18. Vena cava (522)
19. Aorta (522)
20. Esophagus (526)
21. Xiphoid process (515)
22. deceleration injuries (515)
23. parietal (522)
24. visceral (522)
25. Peritonitis (522)
26. umbilicus (522)
27. somatic (522)
28. evisceration (524)
29. oxygen (525)
30. away (530)
31. Breath sounds absent on affected side (519)
32. Distended neck veins (519)
33. Other signs of shock (519)
34. Shifting of trachea away from affected side (519)
35. Visceral pathway (522)
36. Somatic pathway (522)
37. Diffuse (522)
38. Cramping (522)
39. Aching (522)
40. Deformities (Chapter 7, 525)
41. Contusions (Chapter 7, 525)
42. Abrasions (Chapter 7, 525)
43. Punctures or penetrations (Chapter 7, 525)
44. Burns (Chapter 7, 525)
45. Tenderness (Chapter 7, 525)
46. Lacerations (Chapter 7, 525)
47. Swelling (Chapter 7, 525)
48. Patient positioned to minimize any movement of abdomen, usually supine with knees raised and shallow breathing (531)
49. A distended and tense abdomen (531)
50. Abdominal tenderness (531)
51. Abdominal guarding (531)
52. True (516)
53. False (515)
54. False (520)
55. True (516)
56. False (516, 517)
57. True (517)
58. False (520)
59. False (520)
60. True (520)
61. True (520)
62. True (519)
63. False (518)
64. True (521)
65. True (523)

66. False (523)
67. False (523)
68. False (524)
69. False (524)
70. flail chest (516, 517)
71. paradoxical movement (516, 517)
72. pneumothorax or hemothorax (516, 518)

73. rapid extrication (520)
74. supplemental oxygen; stabilization of flail segment (516, 517)
75. d (519)
76. c (519)
77. b (519)
78. a (519)

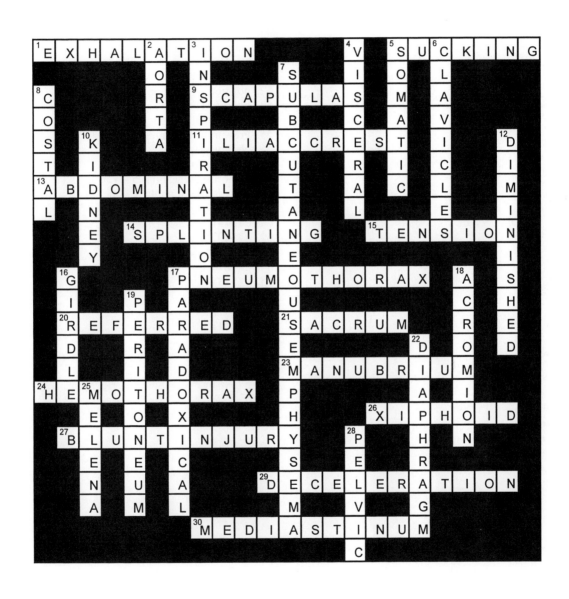

CHAPTER 23

1. a (538)
2. c (538)
3. a (538)
4. b (538)
5. c (538)
6. a (538)
7. b (543)
8. c (543)
9. d (546)
10. b (543)
11. a (548)
12. c (548)
13. c (546)
14. a (544)
15. b (548)
16. c (548)
17. d (539)
18. b (549)
19. b (544, 551)
20. b (547)
21. c (552)
22. d (541)
23. d (548)
24. c (549)
25. d (540)
26. a (549)
27. c (555)
28. b (549)
29. c (541)
30. b
31. b (553)
32. a (538, 539)
33. c (538, 539)
34. b (538, 539)
35. c (544)
36. a (544)
37. b (544)

38. c (549)
39. e (549)
40. a (549)
41. b (549)
42. d (549)
43. c (549)
44. e (549)
45. f (549)
46. b (549)
47. d (549)
48. a (549)
49. paresthesia (548)
50. 10, 15 (562)
51. ischial (558, 559)
52. position of function (551)
53. tibia (541)
54. Reduce pain (548)
55. Prevent further injury (548)
56. Numbness (548)
57. Pain (548)
58. Abnormal sensation (548)
59. Loss of motor ability (548)
60. a (544)
61. c (544)
62. a (549)
63. b (551)
64. d (551)
65. c (538)
66. c (544)
67. a (547)
68. d (551)
69. b (544)
70. a (548)
71. a (548)
72. b (548)
73. b (549)

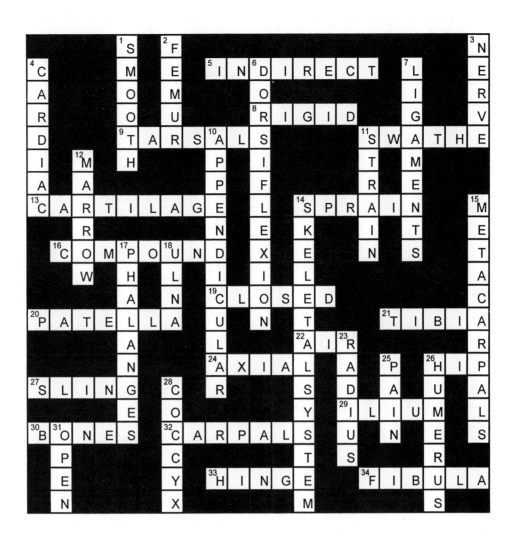

CHAPTER 24

1. a (568)
2. d (568)
3. b (572)
4. d (572)
5. a (572)
6. c (572)
7. b (572)
8. a (572)
9. d (572)
10. a (572)
11. b (570)
12. b (570)
13. b (590)
14. a (571)
15. d (571)
16. a (569)
17. b (569)
18. c (569)
19. c (580)
20. a (580)
21. a (580)
22. c (586)
23. b (583)
24. c (583)
25. b (583)
26. c (583)
27. a (583)
28. a (585, 586)
29. c (586)
30. c (587)
31. b (590)
32. b (587)
33. b (590)
34. c (571-578)
35. a (577-578)
36. b (578)
37. b (579)
38. b (579)
39. a (573)
40. b (573)
41. b (574)
42. b (576)
43. a (593)
44. c (593, 598, 599)
45. b (570)
46. a (570)
47. b (570)
48. a (570)
49. a (570)
50. e (571)
51. a (571)
52. b (571)
53. d (571)
54. c (571)
55. c (571)
56. b (571)
57. a (571)
58. b (568)
59. a (568)
60. c (568)
61. b (569)
62. d (569)
63. a (569)
64. c (569)
65. e (569)
66. a (583, 584)
67. b (583, 584)
68. b (572)
69. c (572)
70. a (572)
71. d (572)
72. c (573)
73. b (573)
74. a (573)
75. c (576)
76. b (592)
77. a (593)
78. b (594)
79. a (594)
80. a (594)
81. Cerebrospinal fluid (571)
82. Clear (571)
83. Fontanel (570)
84. raccoon eyes (583)
85. middle meningeal artery (582)
86. amnesia (583)
87. False (590)
88. True (590)
89. False (593)
90. True (596)
91. False (585)
92. b (585, 586)
93. a (585, 586)
94. a (573, 575)
95. b (579)
96. d (578)
97. b (578)
98. c (583)
99. a (576)
100. c (586)
101. c (586)
102. a (586)
103. b (573)
104. b, a, d, c, f, e (595)

CHAPTER 25

1. b (620)
2. c (605)
3. c (606)
4. a (606)
5. c (606)
6. b (609)
7. d (606)
8. d (606)
9. a (612)

10. c (607)
11. a (607)
12. d (607)
13. b (607)
14. a (607)
15. c (618)
16. c (607)
17. b (607)
18. a (608)
19. c (608)
20. d (610)
21. a (610)
22. c (610)
23. c (610)
24. c (609, 615)
25. a (615)
26. c (615, 616)
27. d (616)
28. d (616)
29. b (616)
30. d (616, 617)
31. c (616)
32. d (627)
33. d (627)
34. d (616, 617)
35. b (627)
36. b (617)
37. d (617)
38. d (617)
39. a (617)
40. a (617)
41. b (615)
42. c (615)
43. b (613)
44. b (613)
45. b (618)
46. b (618)
47. b (619)
48. c (621)
49. c (620)
50. a (609)
51. a (623)
52. c (626)
53. c (623)
54. a (623)
55. d (623)
56. b (623)
57. Grunting (611)
58. Mottling of skin (611)
59. Nasal flaring (611)
60. Retractions (611)
61. Stridor (611)
62. Tachycardia (rapid pulse) (611)
63. Tachypnea (rapid breathing) (611)
64. Wheezing (611)
65. Cyanosis or mottling (611)
66. Fast or slow respiratory rate relative
    to patient's age (611)
67. Little or no air movement (611)
68. Labored breathing and retractions (611)

69. True (611)
70. False (611)
71. True (611)
72. False (619)
73. True (619)
74. False (620)
75. False (612)
76. True (621)
77. c (615)
78. a (615, 616)
79. d (616)
80. b (613)
81. d (608)
82. c (618)
83. b (618, 619)
84. b (615, 616)
85. a (616)
86. b (616)
87. a (616)
88. d (629)
89. a (629)
90. b (629)

CHAPTER 26

1. b (636)
2. a (636)
3. b (636)
4. c (639)
5. d (639)
6. c (638)
7. a (639)
8. a (639)
9. c (639)
10. c (639)
11. b (639)
12. b (639)
13. b (640)
14. d (640)
15. b (640)
16. a (640)
17. c (640)
18. b (641)
19. b (641)
20. d (642)
21. c (635)
22. a
23. c (632)
24. c (632-633)
25. a (632-633)
26. b (632-633)
27. golden hour (643)
28. front (645)
29. d (643)
30. c (644)
31. b (645)
32. b (640)
33. b (642, 643)
34. d (643)

CHAPTER 27

1. b (653)
2. b (651)
3. b (653)
4. c (654)
5. b (655)
6. b (654)
7. c (654)
8. d (650, 651)
9. a (654)
10. a (654)
11. b (651)
12. a (655)
13. a (650)
14. c (650)
15. c (651)
16. d (655)
17. c (655)
18. a (650)
19. c (Chapter 11)
20. b (Chapter 6)
21. c (654)
22. b (655)

CHAPTER 28

1. c (661)
2. a (662)
3. b (669)
4. a (665)
5. a (666)
6. a (668)
7. b (668)
8. c (660)
9. a (669)
10. c (676)
11. c (676)
12. b (676)
13. a (678)
14. d (678)
15. a (670)
16. d (672)
17. b (669)
18. b (678)
19. a (680)
20. c (680)
21. d (680)
22. b (680)
23. d (661)
24. a (661)
25. b (661)
26. c (661)
27. False (664)
28. False (664)
29. True (662, 663)
30. False (663)
31. True (663)
32. False (663)
33. True (667)
34. b (668)
35. a (660)
36. a (669)
37. c (663)
38. a (674, 675)
39. d (674)
40. a (668)
41. c (662)
42. b (670)
43. b (674, 675)
44. d (674)

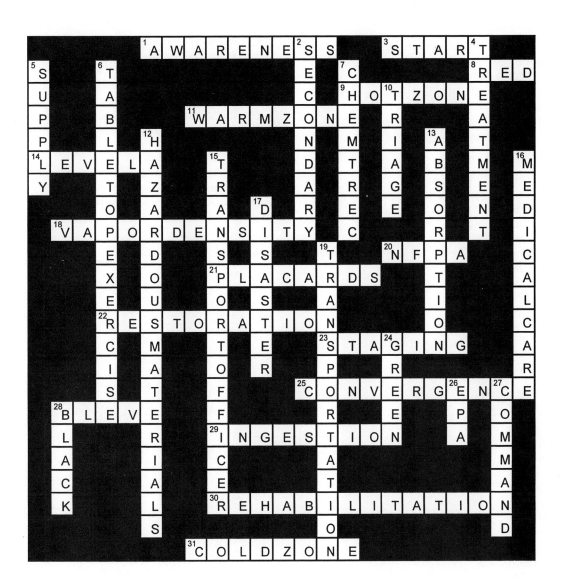

CHAPTER 29

1. b (Chapter 4, Chapter 6)
2. c (Chapter 4, Chapter 6)
3. a (Chapter 4, Chapter 6)
4. b (Chapter 4, Chapter 6, 689)
5. d (Chapter 4, Chapter 6, 688, 690)
6. b (699)
7. d (694, 696)
8. b (688)
9. b (Chapter 4, Chapter 6)
10. b (Chapter 4, Chapter 6)
11. d (Chapter 25)
12. d (Chapter 25, 704)
13. a (Chapter 25, 687)
14. a (Chapter 25)
15. a (Chapter 4, Chapter 6, 693)
16. a
17. d (689)
18. a (703)
19. a (Chapter 4, Chapter 6)
20. d (Chapter 4, Chapter 6)
21. c (690)
22. b (686)
23. a
24. c (Chapter 4, Chapter 6,)
25. a (Chapter 4, Chapter 6, Chapter 14)
26. a (695)
27. b (686, 687)
28. d (687)
29. b (690)
30. d (689)
31. c (691)
32. c (689)
33. a (695)
34. a (695)
35. c (695)
36. b (688)
37. a (690)
38. d (692)
39. a (693)
40. c
41. a (686)
42. c (690)
43. b (689, 695)
44. a (689)
45. b (Chapter 4, Chapter 6)
46. c (Chapter 4, Chapter 6)
47. a (Chapter 4, Chapter 6)
48. f (Chapter 4, Chapter 6)
49. g (Chapter 4, Chapter 6)
50. e (Chapter 4, Chapter 6)
51. d (Chapter 4, Chapter 6)
52. a (691)
53. b (691)
54. b (691)
55. a (691)
56. a (691)
57. b (691)
58. vocal cords (Chapter 4, Chapter 6)
59. alveoli (Chapter 4, Chapter 6)
60. carbon dioxide (Chapter 4, Chapter 6)
61. pharynx (Chapter 4, Chapter 6)
62. Sellick maneuver (687)
63. to 66. Four of the following:
    Prolonged attempts (688)
    Soft tissue trauma (688)
    Right main stem bronchus intubation (688)
    Vomiting (688)
    Slowing of heart rate and induction of
    arrhythmia (688)
    Dislodgement of tube (688)
    Self-extubation (688)
67. False (699)
68. True (689)
69. False (689)
70. True (690)
71. False (690)
72. True (692)
73. True (692)
74. True (687)
75. b
76. c (691)
77. b (690, 704)
78. b (690, 704)
79. c (704)
80. c
81. d
82. c (688)
83. d (688)

CHAPTER 30

1. a (714)
2. a (714)
3. d (716)
4. c (723)
5. c (715, 718)
6. a (722)
7. c (724)
8. b (724)
9. c (724)
10. c (713, 726)
11. d (726)
12. a (728)
13. c (717)
14. b (730)
15. c (728)
16. d (736)
17. d (737)
18. b (730)
19. c (732)
20. d (727)
21. a (728)
22. b (735)
23. a (735)
24. c (735)
25. c (736, 737)
26. d (736, 737)

27. a (736, 737)
28. b (734, 737)
29. multiple casualties, all with the same complaints
    and who were previously well, and at a similar time
    of onset (716)
30. lead (738)
31. safety zone (738)
32. incident command system (717)
33. Recognize a potential NBC event. (714)
34. Take actions to promote the safety of self,
    bystanders, and the victims. (714)
35. Provide medical care. (714)
36. Time (738)
37. Distance (738)
38. Shielding (738)
39. Prevent or minimize transfer of contaminants to an
    internal site. (738)
40. Reduce the amount of radiation dosage from the
    contaminant. (738)
41. Prevent the spread of contamination to other
    persons and areas. (738)
42. False (715)
43. False (715)
44. False (728)
45. False (718)
46. True (718)
47. True (719)
48. False (718)
49. True (722)
50. False (722)
51. True (728)
52. False (734)
53. False (730)
54. True (730)
55. True (731)
56. False (731)
57. False (732)
58. True (737)
59. True (737)
60. True (737)
61. False (740)
62. True (736)
63. True (736)
64. b (738)
65. d (730)
66. c (728)
67. b (728)
68. b (726)

CHAPTER 31

1. c (747)
2. d (750)
3. a (751)
4. c (752)
5. b (753)
6. a (747)
7. a (747)
8. b (747)
9. a (747)
10. b (747)
11. vital capacity (747)
12. stroke volume (747)
13. residual volume (747)
14. arteriosclerosis (747)
15. osteoporosis (747)
16. Problems with sight (749)
17. Problems with hearing (749)
18. Problems in communication (749)
19. Alzheimer's disease (749)
20. Senile dementia (749)
21. Organic brain syndrome (749)
22. Stroke (749)
23. Dry skin turgor (750, 752)
24. Dry oral mucosa (750, 752)
25. Sunken eyes (750, 752)
26. True (752)
27. False (747)
28. True (747)
29. False (748)
30. False (749)
31. c (748)
32. b (751)
33. d (748, 751)
34. b (747)
35. a (752)